CLINICAL
Athletic Training

Edited by

Jeff G. Konin, MEd, ATC, MPT

Lewes Physical Therapy
Lewes, Delaware
Instructor, Physical Therapist Assistant Program
Athletic Trainer
Delaware Technical & Community College
Georgetown, Delaware
President
Coastal Health Consultants, P.A.
Lewes, Delaware

SLACK Incorporated, 6900 Grove Road, Thorofare, NJ 08086-9447

Publisher: John H. Bond
Editorial Director: Amy E. Drummond
Creative Director: Linda Baker

Clinical athletic training/[edited by] Jeff G. Konin
       p. cm.
Includes bibliographical references and index.
ISBN 1-55642-315-2
1. Sports medicine. 2. Athletic trainers. I. Konin, Jeff G.
[DNLM: 1. Physical Education and Training—methods. 2. Allied Health Occupations.
       3. Sports Medicine—methods. QT 255 C641 1996]
RC1210.C585 1996
613.7'11—dc20
DNLM/DLC
for Library of Congress   96-42296

Printed in the United States of America
Published by: SLACK Incorporated
                   6900 Grove Road
                   Thorofare, NJ 08086-9447 USA
                   Telephone: 609-848-1000
                   Fax: 609-853-5991

DEDICATION

To my parents, who encouraged me to follow my dreams.

CONTENTS

ACKNOWLEDGMENTS

Although the didactic material contained in this textbook represents the current ideas and beliefs of the editor and contributors, in reality, the information within is a culmination of the sharing of knowledge, ingenuity, thoughts, and professional skills of many individuals. In particular, I would like to express my deepest appreciation to the following people:

Dave Yeo—my first true mentor in athletic training. While you helped me to branch in the right direction, my journey to seek excellence follows a path back to your wisdom.

Dan Switchenko—for challenging me to be the best that I can be.

Dave Perrin—your guidance, professionalism, and inspiration have helped me to grow as a person, for that I am grateful.

Craig Denegar—your friendship and positive encouragement have led me to believe in myself.

Ethan Saliba—your knowledge and ability to teach will allow me to forever remain a student.

Mike Keirns— for taking me under your wings and explaining to me what the "real world" is all about.

Lance Fujiwara—for helping me through the most difficult times.

Julie Moyer Knowles—a special thank you for providing me with the many opportunities that have enabled me to do what I love most of all.

Joe Gieck—you always said, "At first, do what you think is right, then do what works." Your words have been influential.

Kevin Wilk—the unselfish sharing of your clinical skills enhanced my appreciation for learning.

Chris Arrigo, Ron Berger, Ron Courson, Donna Erber, Cheryl Fuller, Marc Meadows, Johnny Pierce, and Hank Wright—what we shared was special in its own way.

Phil Donley—many thanks for simply taking the time.

Bob Oziomek—the goals and determination that you have instilled in me will remain forever. Keep dreaming.

Joanne Howell—your support, leadership, and encouragement have not gone unnoticed.

James R. Andrews, MD, and *Lawrence Lemak, MD*—for whom I have the utmost respect. You always found time for me, and for that I am extremely grateful.

Mom and Dad—thank you for making the many sacrifices you have made to simply provide me with the opportunities of a lifetime.

All of my students, colleagues, mentors, and athletes—for without all of you, our knowledge and appreciation for the clinical setting would not exist.

The staff at SLACK Incorporated—your assistance and commitment to excellence have been a key driving force behind the motivation to put together a product for which we can all be proud.

Amy Drummond at SLACK Incorporated—for so many things throughout the process of undertaking this project, but, most of all, for believing in me and giving me this opportunity.

Gina, my colleague, my wife, and my best friend—for whom I am the most grateful. You have always been there for me, and that is why I love you.

CONTRIBUTORS

Marjorie J. Albohm, MS, ATC
Director, Sports Medicine and Orthopaedic Research
The Center for Hip and Knee Surgery
Kendrick Memorial Hospital
Mooresville, Indiana

Chris Arrigo, MS, PT, ATC
Clinical Coordinator
Healthsouth Sportsmedicine and Rehabilitation Center
Arlington, Texas

Ronnie P. Barnes, MS, ATC
Head Athletic Trainer
New York Football Giants, Inc.
Founder, Professional Sports Care Management, Inc.
East Rutherford, New Jersey

Dan Campbell, PT/ATC
Manager of Athletic Training Services
University of Wisconsin Hospitals
Sports Medicine Center
Madison, Wisconsin
Past Chair of NATA Governmental Affairs Committee

Jim Clover, MEd, ATC, PTA
Coordinator, The S.P.O.R.T. Clinic
Instructor, Riverside County Office of Education
Riverside Community College
University of California, Riverside
California Baptist College
Riverside, California

Ron Courson, ATC, PT, NREMT
Director of Sports Medicine
University of Georgia Athletic Association
Athens, Georgia

Martin R. Daniel, MS, ATC
Industrial Rehab Consultant
Cass City, Michigan
Healthtrax, Work-Fit Division
Glastonbury, Connecticut

Mark S. De Carlo, MHA, PT, SCS, ATC
Assistant Administrator
Methodist Sports Medicine Center
Indianapolis, Indiana

Phillip B. Donley, MS, PT, ATC
Director, Chester County Orthopedic
and Sports Physical Therapy
Physiotherapy Associates Clinic
West Chester, Pennsylvania

Larry Gardner, ATC, LAT, PT
General Manager of Texas Centers
NovaCare Outpatient Rehabilitation Division
Dallas, Texas

Robert S. Gray, MS, ATC
Coordinator of Athletic Training
Section of Sports Medicine
Cleveland Clinic Foundation
Cleveland, Ohio

Jerome A. "Jai" Isear, MS, PT, ATC
Carolinas Physical Therapy Associates
Charlotte, North Carolina

Michael A. Keirns, PhD, ATC, PT, CSCS
Assistant Professor, Regis University
Denver, Colorado
Director, Excel Physical Therapy
Denver, Colorado

Julie Moyer Knowles, EdD, ATC, PT
President, Pike Creek Sports Medicine Center
Wilmington, Delaware
President, Lewes Physical Therapy
Vice President, Southern Delaware Physical Therapy
Lewes, Delaware

Lyle Knudson, EdD
BIO*Analysis System
Denver, Colorado

Gina Lorence Konin, ATC, PT
Lewes Physical Therapy
Vice President, Coastal Health Consultants, P.A.
Lewes, Delaware

Jeff G. Konin, MEd, ATC, MPT
Lewes Physical Therapy
Lewes, Delaware
Instructor, Physical Therapist Assistant Program
Athletic Trainer
Delaware Technical & Community College
Georgetown, Delaware
President, Coastal Health Consultants, P.A.
Lewes, Delaware

Robert S. Oziomek, MEd, ATC
St. Paul's School
Concord, New Hampshire

Keith J. Webster, MA, ATC
Director of Sports Relations
The Hughston Clinic
Columbus, Georgia

Hank Wright, ATC, PT
Director, Athens Sports Medicine Clinic Inc.
Athens, Georgia

PREFACE

In just a few years, the National Athletic Trainers' Association (NATA) will celebrate its 50th anniversary. To examine the growth that has occurred over this half-century of time would leave one astonished. From the original 200 founding members in 1950 that gathered in Kansas City to the now approximately 7,000 attendees at the annual clinical and symposia, the organization has grown in size and popularity.

Whenever any organization is subject to an expansion and the test of time, change is inevitable. For athletic trainers, this change has presented itself in a number of ways. Educational programs have rapidly progressed to the point of being reviewed and critiqued in an attempt to ensure consistency and competence in one's entry-level skills. Many states have formulated regulatory guidelines that clearly outline the practice of athletic training. In 1990, athletic training was officially recognized by the American Medical Association as an allied health care profession. While not prioritized in the past, athletic trainers are now actively seeking monetary reimbursement from third party payers following the delivery of athletic training services.

One of the biggest areas of change that the profession has come to face revolves around the type of setting in which the athletic trainer delivers his or her services. For many years, one could only find an athletic trainer on the sidelines or in the training room of a collegiate or professional team. This arena of practice has come to be known as the "traditional setting." The traditional setting now has expanded to also include high school athletic training settings. In general, the athletic trainer found him- or herself primarily working with young, healthy athletes who were regularly engaged in competitive activities.

As a result of the demand for athletic health care services, the athletic training profession has found itself in a more diversified position. Not only are the young, healthy athletes seeking the help of athletic trainers, but so also are those physically active, not-so-healthy individuals who wish to receive the same level of professional care that is delivered to the elite athlete. This plea for optimal and equitable treatment has been acknowledged and delivered by those athletic trainers who have braved territorial boundaries to provide quality assistance.

This change and growth in a new era has led to the creation of the "nontraditional setting" and the "nontraditional athletic trainer." Simply put, these terms refer to the athletic trainer who is presently working in a setting other than that previously described. Specifically, the nontraditional setting includes clinical-based facilities, hospitals, corporate offices, and now industrial sites. Realistically, with respect to the athletic trainer, the definition of nontraditional can be expanded to measures where it finds no concrete boundaries other than those imposed by the general assembly.

The NATA has responded to the needs of the general public and the profession. In the late 1980s, a committee was formed to focus on the special concerns of the clinical athletic trainer and those settings that are considered to be nontraditional. This Clinical/Industrial/Corporate Athletic Trainers' Committee continues to be very active and deserves an enormous amount of credit for its insight with respect to the professional growth that has evolved in this area.

In 1992, the entire organization contained approximately 9,000 certified members, of which nearly 34% classified themselves as clinical athletic trainers. Just 4 years later, in 1996, the certified membership grew to nearly 15,000, with approximately 53% of these professionals indicating that they work in an environment that is defined as a clinical setting. This rapid trend for employment in the clinical setting implores us as a profession to adequately prepare ourselves for the ever-changing world of health care delivery.

While we as athletic trainers must continue to hold on to our grass roots and remain proud of our ground-breaking efforts for the care of athletes, we too must recognize our entire potential and capabilities as we endeavor to care for all of those who are considered to be physically active.

The goal of this textbook is to serve as an educational tool in providing the athletic trainer with the necessary knowledge and material that is needed to be successful in the clinical setting. Much of the information within this text has been compiled by the athletic trainers who have proudly yet unselfishly constructed the foundation of clinical athletic training. It is they whose efforts are to be commended and to whom we all owe a great deal of appreciation. For without their intuition, courage, dedication, and persistence, this profession would not be what it is today.

Chapters 1 through 4 discuss the profession of athletic training and are intended to provide the reader with a thorough history of the clinical athletic trainer. To help one better understand how the certified athletic trainer fits into the health care delivery system, various examples of delivery systems are discussed, as is the process of regulating the profession of athletic training. In addition, a chapter has been dedicated to defining the roles and educational backgrounds of those who may work with clinical athletic trainers under a multi-disciplinary approach to health care commonly seen in the clinical setting. It is the firm belief of this author that obtaining a factual understanding of the professional skills and qualifications of those around us promotes teamwork and leads to a facilitation of care.

Chapters 5 through 13 focus on the specific skills and information that not only promote successful employment in the clinical setting, but also prepare one for leadership-type positions. Individual chapters discuss the planning of a new athletic therapy facility, administrative policy and procedure, fiscal management, reimbursement, and clinical marketing. In addition, particular emphasis is placed on the fostering of interpersonal skills. Chapters discussing clinical professionalism, communication, and management styles and approaches are presented as a guide to prepare one for the various routes of professional growth.

Chapters 14 through 20 address practical applications of athletic training and serve as references for common entities that one faces on a daily basis in the clinical setting. The process for taking a thorough and accurate medical history is discussed in detail, as are the accepted methods utilized for proper medical documentation. Furthermore, one of the pioneers of industrial athletic training outlines the critical factors associated with this relatively modern venture. Not wanting to lose focus on the definition of the "traditional versus nontraditional athlete," a chapter is dedicated to those athletes who call for unique methods of care.

The quest into the clinical setting does not come without its share of challenges. One of the biggest tests the athletic trainer will face in this setting is recognizing the associated medical conditions that an athlete or patient may present with other than those that appear to be orthopedically related. An overview of the most common illnesses associated with the various anatomical and physiological systems of the body is reviewed and the implications of each with respect to rehabilitation is clearly explained. As a result of the myriad of pathological states that currently exist, the clinical athletic trainer may also find him- or herself working with a person who has received pharmacological intervention as a means of medical treatment. An introduction to pharmacology and the effect that various commonly used medications have on exercise is summarized in an attempt to prepare the clinical athletic trainer with the educational background necessary to make sound decisions.

Lastly, this text takes an in-depth look at how outcomes assessment plays a vital role in the future of the profession of athletic training. While the process of assessing quality control and performance is not new to many disciplines, it has only been of late that all health care professions are being challenged to justify their worth in the overall delivery of services.

Appendices are included to remind the clinical athletic trainer that the national organization as well as the Clinical/Industrial/Corporate Committee has established guidelines that one can follow when setting personal and professional goals and standards to follow. Also, an appendix has been included to familiarize the reader with the various medical imaging techniques and diagnostic procedures that one may come across while treating persons in the clinical environment.

While this text is in no way all-inclusive of the information utilized in the clinical athletic training setting, it attempts to serve as a foundation for one to incorporate a basis of learning. The many contributors have considerable experience in their respected areas of expertise and have done an excellent job in conveying their thoughts and impressions of how they see the clinical athletic trainer fitting into the profession.

The true test of whether or not one succeeds in the clinical athletic training setting depends on the ability of the individual to utilize his or her skills and adapt to the task at hand. As the legendary coach Vince Lombardi once said, "The dictionary is the only place where success comes before work."

Jeff G. Konin, MEd, ATC, MPT

FOREWORD

Athletic trainers are assuming a more prominent role in the delivery of health care to physically active individuals. Especially noteworthy is the increasing number of athletic trainers being employed in the nontraditional setting. Nontraditional is defined as primarily sports medicine clinics, but also includes hospitals and industrial settings. The National Athletic Trainers' Association (NATA) reports that over the past 5 years, accredited undergraduate and graduate curricula have placed between 20%-30% and 40%-50% of their graduates in this setting, respectively. As of June 1996, the NATA had 14,835 certified members. Forty-two percent of the certified membership was employed in the nontraditional setting. Indeed, when 42% of an organization's membership works in a particular employment setting, the term "nontraditional" would seem inappropriate.

Employment of athletic trainers in sports medicine clinics creates many challenges for the clinician and educator. Many states have failed to legally define the role of the athletic trainer in these settings, which has caused an identity crisis for the practitioner. In fact, in many states athletic trainers cannot identify themselves as such, and must use terms such as "physical therapy aide" to define their role in a clinic. Alumni of my graduate athletic training program at the University of Virginia have expressed consternation over the inability to utilize their talents in evaluation and therapeutic exercise in many sports medicine clinics. I personally have been perplexed that an athletic trainer can legally apply all of the domains of practice in a high school or college athletic training room, but is then restricted from using these same skills in the sports medicine clinic setting.

Athletic trainers employed in the sports medicine clinic setting also treat a wider range of patients, both with respect to age and physical condition. The adage that an athletic injury is an athletic injury, regardless of age or practice setting, is not necessarily true. Providers of health care to older patients face the potential of any number of hidden nonorthopedic conditions. Additionally, it is common to encounter patients who are taking medication, perhaps related to the condition for which they seek treatment, but often totally unrelated. The unrelated medications frequently have the potential to complicate the treatment plan. Thus, an awareness of their presence and an understanding of the potential complications are imperative.

Reimbursement for health care services, and the related importance of clinical documentation and outcomes assessment, have special relevance in the sports medicine clinic setting. Athletic trainers seeking employment as practitioners or personnel managers in a clinic should be well versed in these areas. Interestingly, these issues are having greater relevance to all athletic trainers as the debate about reimbursement for service in traditional practice settings grows.

Jeff Konin, MEd, ATC, MPT, has assembled a distinguished group of professionals to address the aforementioned issues, as well as other matters of importance to athletic trainers in any practice setting. I applaud Mr. Konin for this timely contribution to the athletic training and sports medicine literature. *Clinical Athletic Training* should be required reading for all athletic training students. Athletic training educators should incorporate the subject matter of this text into their curricula. Athletic trainers employed in the sports medicine clinic setting will find *Clinical Athletic Training* both informative and provocative.

David H. Perrin, PhD, ATC
Professor
Curry School of Education
University of Virginia
Charlottesville, Virginia

FOREWORD

It has been a long journey from ancient Greece and Rome to the clinical workplace of the modern athletic trainer. Intriguingly, Herodicus is credited with being the first sports medicine physician and the first athletic trainer. Herodicus would be hard pressed to comprehend the wide duties and responsibilities of today's athletic trainer.

More and more athletic trainers are employed in "nontraditional" settings, such as physical therapy clinics, hospitals, and industrial settings. The goal of this book is to give current and future athletic trainers a better understanding of the knowledge, skills, and attitudes required to succeed in these settings.

During the past 40 years, athletic training has been defined, and it has bloomed as a profession. Modern pioneers such as Jack Hughston, Kenny Howard, Frank McCue, and Joe Gieck, who influenced my personal development, recognized the need for this training and the contributions made by those whose daily concerns are for all aspects of the athlete's health and safety. Like sports medicine, the field of athletic training includes many of the physiological, biomechanical, psychological, and pathological phenomena associated with sports and exercise. The athletic trainer's responsibilities have grown to include clinical application of the work these disciplines perform to improve and maintain functional capacities for sports, exercise, and labor. It also includes prevention and treatment of disease and injuries related to these activities.

In the past decade, the clinical athletic trainer, working with physicians and physical therapists, has taken his or her place in a growing rehabilitation and sports medicine industry. The athletic trainer works alongside the physical therapist delivering modalities of all types in the clinical setting.

In the performance of these clinical duties, athletic trainers have become integral and important members of the rehabilitation team. They expand the influence of physician and therapist while overseeing the application of clinical modalities. They also motivate and build confidence in patients and athletes.

In addition to direct patient care, athletic trainers frequently find themselves faced with a myriad of other duties in the clinical setting. These duties can range from management functions, such as facility and equipment maintenance, to supply, to patient charts and follow-up, to verifying charges, and to cleaning and organizing patient areas. These provide significant challenges to the clinical athletic trainer.

With the development of these diverse and challenging duties in the clinical setting, this book has been designed to help alleviate or minimize the doubts, confusion, and insecurity of ignorance. It addresses in detail the role of the clinical athletic trainer, the role of other healthier providers, the management and administrative aspects of seeing patients in the clinical setting, and it looks at documentation, pharmacology, and outcome-based research.

Assimilation and use of the principles and techniques recorded in this book will give the clinical athletic trainer a great advantage in the clinical or corporate environment. It will help each individual discover more about the fascinating field of clinical athletic training.

James R. Andrews, MD
Medical Director
American Sports Medicine Institute
Birmingham, Alabama

The Role of the Clinical Athletic Trainer

Robert S. Gray, MS, ATC

OBJECTIVES

Upon completion of this chapter, the student will be able to accomplish the following:

1. Appreciate the establishment and history of the Clinical/Industrial/Corporate Athletic Trainers' Committee

2. Be familiar with the domains of athletic training as set forth by the National Athletic Trainers' Association

3. Identify the various settings of employment for nontraditional athletic trainers

4. Recognize the various roles of the clinical athletic trainer

The National Athletic Trainers' Association (NATA) was founded in 1950 by a group of 101 athletic trainers. The expressed purpose of the initial meeting, held in Kansas City, Missouri, was to discuss the concerns and the physical welfare of athletes at colleges, universities, and other institutions. Because of the strong foundation established by these early pioneers, the NATA has grown to well over 20,000 members who dedicate themselves to the care and well-being of the physically active in all settings. The Certified Athletic Trainer (ATC) is a highly qualified health care professional educated to deal with health care problems of today's athletes. ATCs are employed in, but not restricted to the following areas:

- Secondary school interscholastic athletic programs
- Intercollegiate athletic programs
- Professional athletic programs
- Corporate health care programs
- Sports medicine clinics
- Health clubs
- Clinical and industrial health care programs
- Athletic training curriculum programs

The NATA has set competency standards for athletic trainers through the educational system as well as credentialed certification. On June 22, 1990, ATCs were recognized by the American Medical Association (AMA) as "allied health care professionals." Today a certified athletic trainer functions within the five domains of athletic training, set forth by the professional education committee. These domains are: 1) prevention of athletic injuries; 2) recognition, evaluation, and immediate care of athletic injuries; 3) rehabilitation and reconditioning; 4) health care administration; and 5) professional development and responsibility (Table 1-1).

HISTORY OF THE CLINICAL ATHLETIC TRAINER

As a result of the rapid growth of the NATA and the public's emphasis on sports, fitness, and well-being, the employment opportunities for the ATC in nontraditional settings has seen a marked increase. These settings include sports medicine clinics (hospital-based, private, and corporate), corporate programs, industrial programs, and the personal fitness area. Statistics gathered from the annual "Sports Medicine Directory" published by *The Physician and Sports Medicine Journal* indicate a 100% increase in the number of sports medicine facilities nationwide from a period between 1980 and 1990.[1]

In response to this escalating environment, a group of athletic trainers formed what is now known as the Clinical/Industrial/Corporate (C/I/C) Athletic Trainers' Committee of the NATA. The first official meeting of this group took place on June 11, 1988, in Baltimore, Maryland, and was chaired by Roy Don Wilson. The purpose of this meeting was primarily organizational and included the formation of representatives from each district to serve on this committee. The original members who were chosen to serve included Bob Worden, Joe Vegso, John Lopez, Bob Gray, Randy Biggerstaff, Larry Gardner, Carol Kishiyama, Jack Rockwell, John Behrens, and Steve Tollefson.

ROLE OF THE CLINICAL/INDUSTRIAL/CORPORATE ATHLETIC TRAINERS' COMMITTEE

The goals and objectives of the C/I/C committee were initially set forth. These goals included, among others, to educate all of those in the athletic training profession about the evolving role of the clinical athletic trainer, and to protect the interest of this group of athletic trainers within the organization as a whole. At the conclusion of the initial meeting, a list of specific objectives was forwarded to the board of directors of the NATA. These objectives included the following:

1. Increase the number of NATA clinical settings for students to acquire hours toward certification.
2. Request that the board omit geographic limitations necessary to acquire the required internship hours.
3. Appoint a liaison to establish dialogue with the professional education committee, certification committee, ethics committee, and licensure committee to determine if the entry level requirements of the C/I/C athletic trainer were being met.
4. Establish a survey to better assess the needs of the C/I/C ATC.
5. Continue to pursue an accurate and comprehensive list of athletic trainers practicing in C/I/C environments.
6. Establish a dialogue with the members of the sports medicine section of the American Physical Therapy Association (APTA) to discuss areas of mutual concern.
7. To set up district committees consisting of one member from each state.

Following this historic first meeting of the C/I/C committee, much interest was created amongst NATA members. Thus, a second meeting was held and focused on some of the concerns that had been raised regarding the ATCs practicing in C/I/C environments. At the completion of this meeting, the following actions were approved:

1. Each committee member would be responsible for accumulating a list of athletic trainers within their own district who are employed in these type of settings.
2. Each member would accept the following position stand: "The Clinical/Industrial/Corporate Athletic Trainer's Committee is in total support of the NATA's goal of placing ATCs in every high school in the United States."[2]
3. "Any further sponsorship of activities with respect to this group would be channeled through the board of directors of the NATA."[2]

At the conclusion of this meeting, the board of directors also met, at which time they developed a description of the committee. The description of the committee was divided into three sub-categories: composition, purpose, and duties.

The composition of the committee was to be made up from members who are employed in the C/I/C setting. The purpose of the committee was to identify and address issues of concern to athletic trainers in the C/I/C setting and to promote ATCs working in these settings. The duties were two-fold. The first duty was to collect, analyze, and distribute information about the conduct of athletic training in the C/I/C setting. The second duty included the facilitation of communication among ATCs in the C/I/C setting.

Growth of the C/I/C Setting

The C/I/C setting demonstrated a swift growth during the late 1980s and into the early

Table 1-1

Universal Competencies Performance Domains

Universal Competencies	Prevention of Athletic Injuries	Recognition, Evaluation, and Immediate Care of Athletic Injuries	Rehabilitation and Reconditioning of Athletic Injuries	Health Care Administration	Professional Development and Responsibility
Domain-Specific Content	Knowledge and skills particular to each performance domain				
Athletic Training Evaluation	Determination of an athlete's physical readiness to participate	Identification of underlying trauma	Ongoing evaluation of an athlete's progress through various stages of rehabilitation	Documentation of injury status and rehabilitation	Remains up-to-date with current evaluation skills, techniques, and knowledge
Human Anatomy	Normal anatomical structure and function	Recognition of signs and symptoms of athletic injury and illness	Normal anatomical structure and function		Remains up-to-date in current human anatomical research and trends
Human Physiology	Normal physiological functions	Recognition of signs and symptoms of athletic injury and illness	Stages of injury response		Remains up-to-date in current human physiology research and trends
Exercise Physiology	Physiological demand and response to exercise	Recognition of systemic and local metabolic failure	Musculoskeletal and cardiovascular demands placed on the injured athlete		Remains up-to-date with current exercise physiology research and trends
Biomechanics	Normal biomechanical demands of exercise	Identification of pathomechanics	Resolution of pathomechanical motion		Remains up-to-date with current biomechanical research and trends
Psychology/ Counseling	Educational program for the healthy and injured athlete (i.e., alcohol and other drug abuse, performance anxiety)	Recognition of the psychological signs and symptoms of athletic injury and illness	Psychological implications of injury	Communication with, and referral to, the appropriate health care provider	Continues to develop interpersonal and communication skills

Table 1-1 (continued)
Universal Competencies
Performance Domains

Universal Competencies	Prevention of Athletic Injuries	Recognition, Evaluation, and Immediate Care of Athletic Injuries	Rehabilitation and Reconditioning of Athletic Injuries	Health Care Administration	Professional Development and Responsibility
Nutrition	Nutritional demands of the athlete	Recognition of the effects of improper nutritional needs of the competing athlete (i.e., fluid replacement, diabetic shock)	Nutritional demands placed on the injured athlete	Referral to the appropriate health care provider	Remains up-to-date with current nutritional research and trends
Pharmacology	Contraindications and side effects of prescription and nonprescription medications	The role of prescription and nonprescription medications in the immediate/emergency care of athletic injury and illness	The role of prescription and nonprescription medications in the stages of injury response	Proper maintenance and documentation of records for the administration of prescription and nonprescription medication	Remains up-to-date with current knowledge of pharmacological research and trends
Physics	Absorption, dissipation, and transmission of energy of varying materials	The effect of stress loads on the human body (i.e., shear, tensile, compressive forces)	Physiological response to various energies imposed on the body		Remains up-to-date with current knowledge of physics as it relates to athletic training
Organization and Administration	Legal requirements and rules of the sport	Planning, documentation, and communication of appropriate rehabilitation strategies to the necessary parties	Planning, documentation, and communication of appropriate rehabilitation strategies to the necessary parties	Development of operational policies and procedures	Remains up-to-date with current standards of professional practice

Reprinted with permission from the *NATABOC Study Guide Update.*

1990s. A new chairman, John Lopez, was appointed to lead the committee into this era. In response to the rapid growth, the committee submitted the following report to the NATA board of directors following a meeting held in Indianapolis in 1990:

1. The committee would recommend that the board discontinue the NATA approval of allied health clinical settings under the present set-up. Instead, the committee recommends that the individual's respective educational institutions be responsible for approving their own allied clinical setting for students. The committee would provide the necessary guidelines for the selection process.

2. The committee would be responsible for the development of clear cut educational guidelines for athletic training students in the 500 hours allowable within the certification process.

3. The "standards of practice" should be redefined, as they apply to the athletic trainer in this setting.

4. It was strongly recommended that the committee have a voice and input with the "NATA/APTA Task Force." It was also recommended that the task force should not consider that the clinical athletic trainer be utilized in the definition of physical therapist assistants.

5. It was recommended that selected survey results be emphasized regarding the violation of various state laws and practice acts. This survey demonstrated the apparent lack of knowledge toward state laws in athletic training and physical therapy as it pertains to the C/I/C athletic trainers.

6. The C/I/C committee strongly endorses the concept of hiring full-time certified athletic trainers at the high school level and that the clinical athletic trainer only plays a temporary role in this area.

7. The committee would ask for clarification from the board of directors as to what role the committee should be playing for the NATA.

Concerns of the C/I/C Committee

Over the next several years, the C/I/C committee had a very difficult and frustrating task. Direction from the board of directors and the executive director of the NATA as to the role of the committee within the organization was not made terribly clear. The committee's lack of effectiveness, it was felt, was largely due to the result of not having a clearly identified role.

Committee members continued to interact. It was agreed upon that the role of the clinical athletic trainer was quickly changing. And the key to growth in any profession involves the ability to react and respond to change. Unfortunately, it was very difficult for the C/I/C committee to direct itself because its role within the organization was unclear at the time. It became imperative that the committee examine the future of the profession with respect to the ever-changing role of the clinical athletic trainer. The committee as a whole felt that the NATA was initially guilty of benign neglect, in terms of the organization's recognition of the changing role of the clinical athletic trainer as well as the potential impact this change could have on the entire profession. Again, in response to these concerns, the following action items were submitted to the NATA board of directors in 1992 with requests to specifically review each area:

1. Education and role delineation
2. Clinical affiliations
3. Licensure and governmental regulations
4. Professional compliance and ethics

Simply put, the NATA could not afford to allow over 40% of its newly certified athletic trainers who enter the clinical setting for employment to continue to feel a lack of support from the national organization. The committee strongly felt that the national organization must make every effort to recognize individuals in the clinical setting as true allied health professionals, not physical therapy aides, or any other paraprofessional. The athletic trainer could ill afford to be used only as a means of attracting referrals to physical therapy practices. Instead, better utilization of an individual's educational credentials could be established. However, this could not be done without at least the support of his or her own organization and profession.

The C/I/C Athletic Trainer's Committee eventually established a much more recognizable role within the national organization. Thus, the committee continued to grow in efforts, ideas, and importance. In 1992, Robert S. Gray was appointed as the new chairman. Soon thereafter, the following decisions of the committee had been instituted:

1. Set up liaison members with the following committees: high school ATCs, governmental affairs, and professional education.
2. Upon establishment of a liaison relationship between the NATA and the APTA, the NATA would pursue a re-establishment of a Joint Task Force.
3. The board encourages this committee to use its liaison to the Joint Review Committee of Athletic Training and Professional Education to gain implementation of the "Guidelines/Recommendations" for educational institutions to use in selection of allied clinical settings.

Various Roles of the Clinical Athletic Trainer

The evolution of the nontraditional athletic trainer has been exciting and rewarding. While the shift from the traditional setting has led to the establishment and creation of many new employment opportunities, many athletic trainers who find themselves working in clinical, industrial, or corporate settings have taken on the responsibility of various roles. Some of these roles include, but are not limited to, the following:

- Entrepreneurial: owning a facility
- Administrator/Coordinator: being involved in the daily operations of a facility or outreach program
- Marketing Director: marketing the services of an individual's facility to area medical practitioners and the general public. This position would also involve increasing the public's awareness of the services offered by the certified athletic trainer
- Staff Athletic Trainer: treating patients in a facility within the confines of the individual state's practice acts
- Outreach Athletic Trainer: providing athletic training services through contractual obligations to a third-party institution

In addition, a nontraditional athletic trainer may find him- or herself performing a combination of any of the above duties. Not only have our responsibilities changed in the past 25 years with respect to environment, but they have also encouraged us to formulate more accessible services to those who typically have been considered "nontraditional athletes." This group of people includes members of the general public who are physically active but not necessarily involved in competitive sports at the level of registration or scholastic involvement. Likewise, a conscious effort has been made to address the needs of those athletes who are involved in high levels of competition that have not received the highest benefit of services in the past. These athletes include those involved with rodeo and motor sport events, among others.

SUMMARY

Today, the role of clinical athletic trainer is one of variety and opportunity. The student must be prepared with a well-rounded education and a wide assortment of clinical experiences. In addition to being able to competently treat athletic injuries, an athletic trainer in this day and age must possess a keen knowledge of management skills, fiscal responsibility, clinical marketing, reimbursement, and documentation, among other crafts that require an individual to successfully practice in the clinical, corporate, or industrial athletic training setting.

As a result of the changes in the health care industry, the certified athletic trainer must also be familiar with functional outcomes and the role that he or she has with respect to modifications of treatment and services. The athletic trainer must be able to measure the quality of care that is delivered in the nontraditional setting in order to successfully assess the functional restoration of a person's underlying condition, and more importantly, to develop a team approach among allied health professionals. Multidisciplinary approaches to treatment within C/I/C environments include the services of a certified athletic trainer and are established through educational backgrounds, state laws, and professional communication and interaction skills.

Study Questions

1. Discuss how the domains of athletic training pertain to you in your present role.
2. Explain how the establishment of the "nontraditional" or clinical athletic trainer differs from the "traditional" athletic trainer.
3. List the various roles and responsibilities of the clinical athletic trainer.
4. If you were serving as a member of the Clinical/Industrial/Corporate Athletic Trainer's Committee, what issues would you feel are important to address as they might play a role with respect to the clinical athletic trainer and the profession of athletic training as a whole? How would you suggest these concerns be handled?

References

1. Sports medicine directory 1990. *Physican and Sportsmedicine.* 1990;18(9):SSE3-SS34.

2. Minutes from the annual meeting of the Clinical/Industrial/Corporate Athletic Trainers' Committee, Dallas, Texas. June 1989.

Suggested Readings

ATCs in the clinical setting. *NATA News.* January 1993:16–19.

Gray, RS. Why the clinical athletic trainer? *NATA News.* January 1993:22.

Membership Snapshot: ATCs in the clinical Setting. *NATA News.* January 1993:20.

The Roles of Allied Health Care Providers

Jeff G. Konin, MEd, ATC, MPT

OBJECTIVES

Upon completion of this chapter, the student will be able to accomplish the following:

1. Distinguish among primary, secondary, and tertiary health care providers

2. Define and explain the process of accreditation

3. Define and explain the process of regulation of health care providers

4. Identify the various members involved in allied health care

5. Identify the roles and responsibilities of allied health care providers

The task of providing competent and efficient care to an individual has become quite complex. No longer is it recognized that one single individual possesses the expertise in rendering care to an athlete. Instead, many people may play a role in the delivery of care. The expanding role of health care providers has been brought to light for many reasons: 1) the advancement of medical technology, 2) the improvements of evaluative skills, 3) the results of short- and long-term research, and 4) the resultant ongoing changes in health care delivery systems.

Although the role of the certified athletic trainer has expanded to meet the needs of these changes, so have the roles of many other health professionals. It is incumbent upon the athletic trainer to recognize the role that each of these individuals play in the delivery of care. It is also important for the athletic trainer to understand how he or she fits into this system, thus providing for an optimal team approach. Understanding, recognizing, and respecting each other's roles and responsibilities may ultimately lead to the best care for an athlete.

DESIGNATION OF PROVIDERS

Allied health care providers can be subdivided into one of three categories depending on the type of care that they render. These categories are primary, secondary, and tertiary care providers.[1]

A primary care provider typically is the person who provides the first intervention for an individual who is seeking medical attention. The primary care provider is often referred to as a direct provider of care. Although in many instances the athletic trainer is the very first person to assess a situation, a physician is more commonly recognized as the primary care provider in the clinical setting. Within the health care system, the physician who serves as a primary care provider may be specially trained in areas such as general practice, pediatrics, or internal medicine.

Those who need further medical attention beyond that of a primary care level alone may seek the skills of a secondary care provider. A provider of secondary care is not necessarily one who is trained above and beyond the level of a primary care provider. Instead, a provider of secondary care simply renders services, equipment, and/or testing procedures that are not readily available at the primary care level. A secondary care provider who makes available certain products or services that enable a primary care provider to meet the needs of an individual is called an *indirect provider*. Orthotists, radiologic technicians, surgical technicians, and phlebotomists are examples of allied health care professionals who operate at a secondary level of care.

An individual who receives treatment in the form of tertiary care is said to be in a facility that has the necessary resources to provide all aspects of care within its center. Tertiary care facilities typically provide both primary and secondary levels of care on-site, and serve as a regional center for other community-based hospitals that do not have the full privilege of resources available within their own settings.

ACCREDITATION OF HEALTH CARE PROVIDERS

With the availability of various providers possessing unique skills and disciplines, it is important to maintain a minimal level of standard of care. This is accomplished in one form through the process of accreditation. To accredit is to recognize the meeting and maintaining of standards that would enable an individual to receive a certificate or registration in a certain domain.

For example, when an individual graduates from an NATA approved curriculum, that person is graduating from an institution that has been accredited according to the national standards set by the governing body of accreditation for athletic trainers. Physicians, physical therapists, nurses, and many other health care providers have similar educational accrediting processes in place to ensure that each curriculum meets the minimum requirements necessary for a graduate to enter the field as a professional.

Individual professions are not alone in the policing of their graduates. The task of providing competent health care with appropriate standards of care is an ongoing process. Therefore, facilities such as hospitals are required to undergo regular evaluations to determine if they are meeting the criteria set forth to provide sound care. Whether in a curricular or hospital-based setting, it is essential to maintain certain levels of consistency within the delivery of health care. Doing so helps to ensure safe and competent care.

REGULATION OF HEALTH CARE PROVIDERS

In addition to implemented policies by professionals to instill adequate levels of performance within their own ranks, the government has also taken an active role in the process of regulating health care providers. Regulation is the process of enacting a rule or law in an attempt to bring order, method, or uniformity to an issue.[2] Regulation may or may not be directed toward any individual profession per se, and it can be adopted at both federal and state levels.

At the federal level public health care policies have been long instituted to ensure that certain guidelines are followed. For example, to be considered as an approved provider for medicare services, facilities must comply with all of the requirements set forth by the federal government. These requirements may range from the accessibility of a facility for individuals with disabilities to the types of solutions that are used to sterilize equipment.

Because many institutions rely heavily on federal funds, these institutions must also comply with the requirements and standards that are outlined by the governing agencies of the federal government.

Legislation at the state level is inclusive only in the jurisdiction set forth and relates to services provided in the confines of the said state only. Legislation at the state level is often designed primarily to protect the members of the community from rising health care costs by controlling the revenues and expenditures of the providers.

Local legislation is also enacted for the purposes of establishing licensure, registration, and rules and regulations for the many different providers of health care. This aids in protecting the skills and services of a particular profession from infringement by otherwise unlicensed/unregistered and nonqualified individuals.

ROLES AND RESPONSIBILITIES

It is clear that many different health professions exist these days. Ultimately, the common goal of each provider is to ensure that the consumer receives the highest level of care and returns to an uncomplicated level of function. In the clinical setting, this function may range from professional tennis to intramural softball. Regardless, each player on the health team has a role and responsibility.

An athletic trainer must understand that his or her role in the provision of care is essential to his or her success. Just as important is understanding the roles of the other health care providers. Many providers have skills that are inclusive to their formal educational and clinical training. However, other providers possess skills that are not inclusive to their training, and in fact may be shared by other providers. Thus, a team approach to treatment is most beneficial.

In order to better appreciate the role of each provider, this next section outlines the roles and responsibilities, as well as the educational requirements of the various members of the health care team that an athletic trainer may interact with during the delivery of care.

Physicians examine patients, obtain medical histories, perform and interpret diagnostic tests, diagnose illnesses, and administer treatment. There are two types of physicians: a Doctor of Medicine (MD) and a Doctor of Osteopathy (DO). Although both may use all accepted methods of treatment, such as drug therapy and surgery, DOs generally place special emphasis on the body's musculoskeletal system.[3]

Most MDs specialize in one area of medicine. Table 2-1 represents a distribution of these areas as researched by the AMA.

Table 2-1
Percentage of Physicians by Specialty

General and Family Practice 11.0

Medical Specialties

Allergy	0.5
Cardiovascular diseases	2.5
Dermatology	1.2
Gastroenterology	1.2
Internal medicine	16.7
Pediatric cardiology	0.2
Pediatrics	6.9
Pulmonary diseases	1.0

Surgical Specialties

Colon and rectal surgery	0.1
General surgery	6.0
Neurological surgery	0.7
Obstetrics and gynecology	5.4
Ophthalmology	2.5
Orthopedic surgery	3.2
Otolaryngology	1.3
Plastic surgery	0.7
Thoracic surgery	0.3
Urological surgery	1.4

Other Specialties

Aerospace medicine	0.1
Anesthesiology	4.3
Child psychiatry	0.7
Diagnostic radiology	2.6
Emergency medicine	2.4
Forensic pathology	0.1
General preventive medicine	0.2
Neurology	1.5
Nuclear medicine	0.2
Occupational medicine	0.4
Pathology	2.6
Physical medicine and rehabilitation	0.7
Psychiatry	5.6
Public health	0.3
Radiation oncology	0.5
Radiology	1.2
Other specialty	1.5
Unspecified/unknown/inactive	12.6

Source: American Medical Association.

All states, the District of Columbia, and the U.S. territories require physicians to be licensed. Licensure requirements for both DOs and MDs include graduation from an accredited medical school, completion of a licensing examination, and anywhere between 1 and 7 years of graduate medical education. Graduate medical education is performed in the area of residencies and internships. Physicians who seek board certification in a specialty area will undergo additional clinical training.

Physician Assistants serve to support a physician in the performing of tasks such as medical history taking, patient examination, ordering and interpreting laboratory tests and x-rays, and treating minor injuries via such methods as suturing, splinting, and casting. Physician Assistants must always work under the supervision of a physician, which may be defined differently in each state.[3]

Most states require some form of licensure or certification that must be preceded by the graduation from an accredited institution. Upon completion of an examination, an individual receives the credentials PA-C, representing a Physician Assistant-Certified.

Dentists prevent, diagnose, and treat the teeth and tissues of the mouth. Dentists may perform surgery and administer and prescribe medications.[3]

All 50 states and the District of Columbia require dentists to be licensed. Candidates must graduate from a dental school accredited by the American Dental Association's Commission on Dental Accreditation and pass written and practical examinations to qualify for licensure. Most dental schools award either the degree of Doctor of Dental Surgery (DDS) or Doctor of Dental Medicine (DMD).

Podiatrists diagnose and treat disorders, diseases, and injuries of the foot and ankle. This includes the treatment of calluses, bunions, heel spurs, and ligament sprains. Podiatrists may use medications, order x-rays and laboratory tests, and perform surgery when appropriately trained.[3]

All 50 states and the District of Columbia require a license for the practice of podiatric medicine. An individual must be a graduate of an accredited college of podiatric medicine and pass written as well as oral examinations to qualify. Many states also require the completion of an additional residency program. Graduates of accredited programs receive the Doctor of Podiatric Medicine degree (DPM).

Podiatrists may specialize in areas such as surgery, public health, and orthopedics, to name a few. A podiatrist must be certified by the American Board of Podiatric Surgery, the American Board of Podiatric Public Health, or the American Board of Podiatric Orthopaedic and Primary Podiatric Medicine to be recognized as a specialist.

Chiropractors diagnose and treat patients whose health problems are associated with the body's muscular, nervous, and skeletal systems, especially the spine. Chiropractors believe that misalignment of spinal vertebrae or irritation of the spinal nerves can alter many important bodily functions by affecting the nervous system. Chiropractors use natural, drugless, nonsurgical health treatments and rely on the body's inherent recuperative abilities.[3]

All states regulate the practice of chiropractors and grant licenses to chiropractors who meet educational requirements and pass a state board examination. Most states' licensing boards require completion of a 4-year chiropractic college course following at least 2 years of undergraduate education. All state boards recognize academic training in chiropractic colleges accredited by the Council on Chiropractic Education, which grants the degree of Doctor of Chiropractic (DC).

Pharmacists dispense drugs that are prescribed by physicians and other health practitioners and provide information to patients about the medications. Pharmacists may advise on issues such as selection of a medication, dosage, and side effects.[3]

All states, the District of Columbia, and U.S. territories require a license to practice pharmacy. A pharmicist must graduate from an accredited college of pharmacy, pass a state examination, and serve a supervised internship under a licensed pharmacist to qualify for a license. Programs are accredited by the American Council on Pharmaceutical Education. Most pharmacists possess a bachelor of science in pharmacy, while some further their education and obtain a Doctor of Pharmacy (PharmD).

Optometrists examine people's eyes to diagnose vision problems and eye disease. Optometrists test for visual acuity, depth and color perception, and coordination of the eyes, among other areas. Optometrists may prescribe eyeglasses, contact lenses, vision therapy, and low vision aids. In many states, they can use topical and oral medications to evaluate and treat eye injuries.[3]

All 50 states and the District of Columbia require that all optometrists be licensed. A candidate must earn a Doctor of Optometry (OD) degree from an accredited optometry school and pass both a written and a clinical state board examination to qualify.

Ophthalmologists are physicians who diagnose and treat eye injuries and diseases. They may perform surgery and prescribe medications, eyeglasses, and contact lenses.[3]

Physical Therapists improve the mobility, relieve the pain, and prevent or limit permanent physical disabilities of patients with injury or disease through the intervention of patient education, exercise, and therapeutic modalities. Some physical therapists treat a wide variety of conditions, while others specialize in areas such as pediatrics, orthopedics, and neurology.[3]

All 50 states and the District of Columbia require a physical therapist to be licensed. A candidate must be a graduate of an accredited physical therapy program as recognized by the Commission on Accreditation in Physical Therapy Education (CAPTE) and pass a nationally administered written examination. Currently, there is a shift from 4-year bachelor programs to 2-year entry level master programs. In addition, many postgraduate degrees may be obtained in physical therapy, and the profession recognizes 19 areas in which specialization can be achieved through certification (Table 2-2).

Physical Therapist Assistants also administer physical therapy care and must graduate from an accredited 2-year institution. However, not all states have licensure for PTAs and therefore the scope of practice may vary from state to state. PTA education does not include evaluative skills, and although in many states PTAs may perform treatments without direct on-site supervision of a physical therapist, physical therapist assistant edu-

---

Table 2-2
APTA Specialty Sections

Acute Care	Geriatrics	Pediatrics
Administration	Hand Rehabilitation	Private Practice
Aquatic Physical Therapy	Health Policy, Legislation,	Research
Cardiopulmonary	and Regulation	Sports Physical Therapy
Clinical Electrophysiology	Neurology	Veterans Affairs
Community Home Health	Oncology	Women's Health
Education	Orthopedics	

cation is directed with the primary focus of assisting a physical therapist.

Occupational Therapists help individuals with mentally, physically, developmentally, or emotionally disabling conditions to develop, recover, or maintain daily living and work skills.[3]

The minimal educational requirement to become an occupational therapist is a bachelor's degree, although many programs are offered as entry-level master's programs. Presently, all states and the District of Columbia require a license to practice occupational therapy. A candidate must graduate from an accredited program and pass a national certification examination given by the American Occupational Therapy Certification Board.

Occupational Therapy Assistants may also become certified (COTA) to treat similar caseloads as the occupational therapist. Most schools that offer this type of a program require 2 years of education, whereas the limitations of the scope of practice are defined on a state-wide basis.

Social Workers help individuals cope with problems that may interfere with rehabilitation such as inadequate housing, unemployment, lack of job skills, financial management, serious illness, disability, substance abuse, unwanted pregnancy, or antisocial behavior. Social workers work closely with families and significant others to create a system of support for the individual being treated.[3]

A bachelor's degree (BSW) is the minimum requirement for most social workers. However, in health care settings, a master's degree in social work (MSW) is generally necessary.

Nutritionists plan nutritional programs to aid in the prevention of illness, promote healthy eating habits, and to optimize performance. They are otherwise known as dieticians.[3]

Over 50% of the states in this country currently have laws governing the area of dietetics. The Commission on Dietetic Registration of the American Dietetic Association (ADA) awards the Registered Dietician (RD) to those who pass a certification exam after completing their academic education and supervised experience. The minimal educational requirement is a bachelor's degree with a major in areas such as dietetics or nutrition.

Registered Nurses (RN) provide for the physical, mental, and emotional needs of patients through evaluation, assessment, planning, and implementation. Registered nurses provide care to include examinations, treatments, and the administration of medications.[3]

Although RNs are governed by individual state laws, responsibilities will vary from one work site to another. All states do require that the candidate graduate from an accredited institution (as approved by the state boards of nursing), as well as pass a national licensing examination. The educational background in terms of years varies among a diploma program, an associate's degree (ADN), and a bachelor's of science degree in nursing (BSN).

Licensed Practical Nurses provide nursing services under the direction of various professionals, including physicians and registered nurses. LPNs may take vital signs, help with personal hygiene, administer prescribed medications, and start intravenous fluids in certain states.[3]

Most practical nursing programs are 1 year in length and must be state approved. An LPN must pass a licensing examination issued by the National Council of Licensure Examinations (NCLEX) to practice.

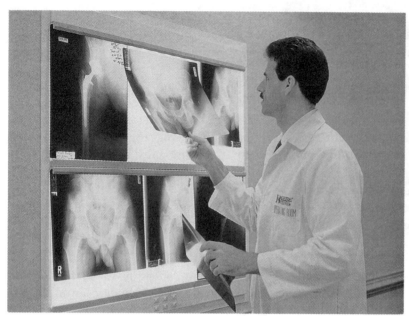

Figure 2-1. Radiologic technologists operate equipment utilized for diagnostic procedures.

Advanced Practice Nurses are registered nurses who have advanced education in the assessment of the physical and psychosocial health–illness status of individuals, families, or groups in a variety of settings through health and development, history-taking, and physical examination. APNs may include nurse practitioners and midwives among others.[4]

A registered nurse, who possesses a BSN, can work as an APN. Licensure is also required for both APN and RN.

Respiratory Therapists evaluate, treat, and care for patients with breathing disorders or illnesses. Evaluations include testing the capacity of the lungs as well as analyzing the levels of oxygen availability.[3]

Forty-two states now maintain licensure for respiratory therapists. In addition, the National Board of Respiratory Care issues credentials for Certified Respiratory Therapy Technicians (CRTT) and Registered Respiratory Therapists (RRT). The candidate must graduate from an accredited 1-, 2-, or 4-year program recognized by the Commission on Accreditation for Allied Health Education Programs (CAAHEP) to qualify.

Speech Therapists/Audiologists assess and treat people with speech, language, voice, and fluency disorders and those with hearing disorders, respectively.[3]

Forty-three states regulate practice, and all require a minimum of a master's degree, supervised clinical experience, passing of a nationally administered examination, and 9 months of post-graduate professional experience.

Radiologic Technologists operate equipment utilized for diagnostic procedures that use x-radiation, high-frequency ultrasound, magnetic fields, and radioactive isotopes. Radiographers practice under the supervision of physicians.

Educational programs range from 2 to 4 years in length and may lead to certificates or associate's or bachelor's degrees. Programs may be sponsored by hospitals, colleges, or technical institutes, and each must be accredited by the Joint Review Committee on Education in Radiologic Technology (JRCERT). With additional training, radiologic technologists may become specialists in such areas as ultrasound, computerized tomography, magnetic resonance imaging, nuclear medicine, and radiation therapy (Figure 2-1).

Exercise Physiologists work with athletes and patients to improve cardiovascular components of exercise. Exercise physiologists emphasize prevention and maintenance, but are also involved with treatment following injury or illness.

Most exercise physiology educational programs are offered as 4-year bachelor's degrees. However, many exercise physiologists go on to obtain master and doctorate level degrees.

Strength and Conditioning Specialists work primarily on the strength and conditioning components of athletes and the general population. Strength and conditioning specialists receive a certification (CSCS) from the National Strength and Conditioning Association (NSCA) following the completion of a bachelor's degree and the passing of a written and practical nationally administered examination.

Massage Therapists, through the art of various forms of massage, attempt to produce physical, mental, and emotional changes via soft tissue manipulation.[4]

The education of a massage therapist can vary from one institution to another. Overall, 55 schools in the United States are accredited or approved by the American Massage Therapy Association (AMTA), which requires at least 500 hours of classroom instruction and at least 300 hours in massage theory and technique. Licensure requirements, if any, also differ from one state to another, with some states requesting additional hours of instruction prior to application.

Emergency Medical Technicians (EMTs) provide immediate care and transport injured individuals to medical facilities. Depending on the level of training, EMTs may perform interventions such as opening airways, controlling bleeding, treating for shock, administering oxygen, immobilizing fractures, and assisting in childbirth. Advanced training would allow a technician to administer intravenous fluids and use defibrillators in emergency situations.[4]

Basic EMT training includes 100–120 hours of classroom work plus 10 hours of internship in a hospital emergency room. Advanced training courses vary in depth. Graduates of approved EMT-basic training programs who pass a written and practical examination administered by the state certifying agency or the National Registry of Emergency Medical Technicians earn the title Registered EMT-Basic.

It is clear that a person may come across any of the above mentioned professionals during the course of treatment. In order to provide optimal care, it is imperative that team approaches be taken to best utilize the skills of all of those involved in the implementation of care. It is essential for athletic trainers to understand the roles and responsibilities of the members of the team to effectively perform in an interactive multidisciplinary approach. Additional information about these professions can be obtained from their respective national organizations. (See Additional Resources at the end of this chapter.)

SUMMARY

The role of athletic trainers has expanded to incorporate care in the clinical setting along with many other allied health care providers. These health care providers are typically referred to as primary, secondary, and tertiary care providers. The type of service and intervention with a patient determines the classification of the provider.

Health care facilities and professions are accredited by different organizations to ensure that a minimal standard of care is being delivered. These health care facilities and professions are regulated by different governing bodies to further establish a policy of the delivery of care. This is often done through a set of rules and regulations at the federal and state levels.

Each health care provider has been trained to deliver a specific type of care to an individual. It is not uncommon to see more than one profession overlapping its skills. In an attempt to provide optimal care in a clinical setting, it is best to utilize a team approach by incorporating various disciplines in the rendering of care to an individual.

Study Questions

1. Identify the reasons for the expanding role of health care providers.
2. List and define the three types of health care providers.
3. Give examples of situations in a clinical setting in which an athletic trainer might interact with the different levels of health care providers.
4. Define accreditation and explain its role in athletic training.
5. Discuss the process of regulation. Give one example of how your state's rules and regulations affect your practice.
6. List all of the allied health care providers and their roles with a team approach for each of the following conditions: a) low back pain, b) anorexia nervosa, c) left ventricular hypertrophy, d) corneal abrasion, e) talus fracture, f) grade II knee sprain, and g) pneumothorax.

References

1. Nosse LJ, Friberg DG. *Management Principles for Physical Therapists*. Baltimore, Md:Williams & Wilkins;1992.

2. *Webster's New Collegiate Dictionary*. Springfield, Mass:Merriam-Webster Inc, Publishers; 1994.

3. US Department of Labor, Bureau of Labor Statistics. Washington, DC:US Government Printing Office;1994–1995.

4. Hopke WE. *Encyclopedia of Careers and Vocational Guidance*, 9th ed. Chicago, Ill:JG Ferguson Publishing Co.;1993.

Additional Resources

Allied Health Education Directory, 22nd Edition. American Medical Association, Chicago;1994-1995.

American Academy of Physician Assistants, 950 North Washington St., Alexandria, VA 22314.

American Association for Respiratory Care, 11030 Ables Lane, Dallas, TX 75229-4593.

American Association of Colleges of Pharmacy, 1426 Prince St., Alexandria, VA 22314-2841.

American Association of Dental Schools, 1625 Massachusetts Ave., NW, Washington, DC 20036.

American Chiropractic Association, 1701 Clarendon Blvd., Arlington, VA 22209.

American Dental Trade Association, SELECT Program, 211 East Chicago Avenue, Suite 1804, Chicago, IL 60611.

American Dietetic Association, 216 West Jackson Blvd., Chicago, IL 60606-6995.

American Massage Therapy Association, 820 Davis Street, Suite 100, Evanston, IL 60201-4444.

American Medical Association, 515 North State St., Chicago, IL 60610.

American Nurse's Association, 600 Maryland Ave, SW, Washington, DC 20024-257.

American Occupational Therapy Association, P.O. Box 1725, 1383 Piccard Drive, Rockville, MD 20849-1725.

American Optometric Association, Educational Services, 243 North Lindbergh Blvd, St. Louis, MO 63141-7881.

American Osteopathic Association, Department of Public Relations, 142 East Ontario St., Chicago, IL 60611.

American Physical Therapy Association, 1111 North Fairfax St., Alexandria, VA 22314.

American Society of Radiologic Technologists, 15000 Central Ave, SE, Albuquerque, NM 87123-3917.

Commission on Accreditation of Allied Health Education Programs, 515 North State Street, Suite 7530, Chicago, IL 60610.

Council on Chiropractic Education, 7975 N. Hayden Road, Suite A-210, Scottsdale, AZ 85258.

National Association for Practical Nurse Education and Service, Inc., 1400 Spring St., Suite 310, Silver Spring, MD 20910.

National Association for Social Workers, 750 First St., NE, Suite 700, Washington, DC 20002-4241.

National Strength and Conditioning Association, PO Box 38909, Colorado Springs, CO 80937.

Acknowledgments

Special thanks to Junior Gray, MBA, RT(R), Anne Lawton, OTR/L, James G. Little, MEd, CPFT, RRT, David C. Ludema, MA, RT(R), Mara Schmittinger, OTR/L, and June Turansky, MSN, RN, for their assistance in the preparation of this chapter.

CHAPTER 3

Regulation of Athletic Training

Dan Campbell, PT/ATC
Jeff G. Konin, MEd, ATC, MPT

OBJECTIVES

Upon completion of this chapter, the student will be able to accomplish the following:

1. Describe the history of the regulatory process of athletic trainers

2. Identify and define the various types of legislative regulation to include licensure, certification, registration, and exemption

3. Recognize the common parameters that define the scope of practice for an athletic trainer under regulation

4. Discuss the challenges involved with regulation of athletic training

Regulation of athletic training, while probably on the minds of several individual athletic trainers, did not receive attention from the leadership of the NATA until 1976. Frank George, President of the NATA at that time, convened a meeting of concerned athletic trainers in Chicago. His fear lay grounded in the rumor that athletic trainers may be exposed to criminal action if those athletic trainers performed modality treatments for injuries of athletes. Use of treatment modalities, such as ultrasound or diathermy, were limited in many states to those individuals licensed to practice physical therapy. Athletic trainers who performed those types of treatments without having either an order from the team physician or actually having the team physician on the premises supervising the treatments were especially vulnerable to violation of a physical therapy practice act.

The nascent national certification process offered by the NATA could not be relied on as a protective mechanism because it had not been tested for this consideration in the courts. Furthermore, George felt that athletic trainers were in danger of losing employment.

The state of Texas had enacted the only licensing bill for athletic trainers (1971), although Illinois and Kentucky were trying to gain regulation at the time. Even though Texas was unable to give proof of protection of employment, the mechanism of state regulation held attractive qualities. Regulation could present a definition of athletic training, elucidate a scope of practice, provide recognition for the profession, and most importantly, protect athletes from harm due to poorly educated or untrained practitioners. The emphasis of the Chicago meeting was to determine a method through which the NATA could assist its members in solidifying their role in the health care of athletes and thus ensure their own employment.[1]

A short time later, the NATA Board of Directors formed a "licensure committee." This committee was charged with the task of serving as a resource for athletic trainers who wished to pursue regulation within their own states. This included the establishment of a "model legislative act." Twenty years after this humble beginning, 35 states (and the District of Columbia) enjoy some form of regulation of the practice of athletic training. However, because each state is a sovereign entity, each state's athletic training practice act is unique. Athletic trainers are well-advised to know their state practice act and not to assume that the practice parameters of athletic training are the same in every state. Throughout the discussion of regulation in this text, it is important for the reader to recollect the fact that each state may define the terms of various types of regulation differently.

TYPES OF LEGISLATIVE REGULATION

Licensure

Each state sets its own level of practice competency for any regulated profession. Licensure is the strongest form of public protection afforded by a legislature. Through licensure, the state limits the number of practitioners. The state can set those types of limits by dictating that only individuals who have met specific educational or training requirements can apply for a title, or can perform functions that are restricted to licensed individuals through the language of the act itself. Table 3-1 represents a list of the states that currently have licensure.

Table 3-1
States that License Athletic Training

Alabama	Iowa	Ohio
Arkansas	Maine	Oklahoma
Delaware	Massachusetts	Rhode Island
Florida	Mississippi	South Dakota
Georgia	Nebraska	Texas
Illinois	New Mexico	
Indiana	North Dakota	

Often the educational requirements alone are prohibitive for many applicants. Criteria of a baccalaureate degree with defined courses of major studies or additional internship hours are common methods for limiting the pool of applicants. It is easy to see how setting higher educational thresholds can limit applicants to those wealthy enough to afford long-term preparation.

Defining acceptable internship experience parameters can also restrict the number of applicants for a license. By narrowly defining the types of sites, level of supervision necessary or qualifications of supervisors, it is possible to control the internship experience. Conceivably, each applicant would be competing for one of relatively few positions as an intern. In addition, supervisory agencies that administer the act can set rules and regulations that also limit the number of practitioners.

Applicants may need to meet criteria of "good moral character," show absence of a criminal record, or procure letters of recommendation from currently licensed practitioners as part of the application process. Failure to meet all criteria for application would eliminate that applicant from being able to obtain the certificate of regulation.

The supervising agency also determines the type of examination needed to winnow out less qualified applicants. Even though the agency may designate a common (or national) professional examination instead of writing its own examination, the agency sets its own minimal passing score. In that way, each state maintains its sovereignty in protecting its citizens while at the same time accepting a common method. In addition, the movement of licensed practitioners from one state to another is not hindered and the state does not need to bear the cost of offering frequent examinations for a small pool of applicants.

Licensure may tend to be somewhat expensive. A state may enact a tariff from practitioners in the form of license fees, at which time a practitioner may be required to pay these fees in order to maintain an updated license. Failure to pay these fees may result in a loss of a license and subsequent inability to practice the profession in a given state.

Licensed professionals tend to be expensive for the purchaser as well. Many licensed professionals charge a fee for their services to recover the costs of a license as well as to regain educational costs. Remember, though, that licensure assures the public that an individual has met state requirements to practice the profession and therefore reduces the risk to public safety.

The supervisory agency usually has the responsibility of monitoring actions of licensed individuals to ensure that only allowable functions, as delineated in the law, are performed by the practitioners. The supervisory agency also has the responsibility of preventing unlicensed individuals from performing functions that are limited to the licensed practitioner.

The state does not often recognize titles as necessarily being discriminatory and will look to the functions performed by the individual as the standard for violation of a professional practice act.

For an example in the sports medicine realm, consider the unregulated individual who calls him- or herself a "sports medicine specialist" and performs functions delineated in the athletic training practice act. Unless given specific exemption from the practice act, that individual is liable for prosecution if the state applies the "duck" standard. That is, if it looks like a duck, waddles like a duck, quacks like a duck, has feathers and a bill like a duck, then it's a duck until proven otherwise. In other words, the title of "sports medicine specialist," even if not defined in the law, and even though the individual is performing functions commonly associated with the title, does not give that individual the ability to perform the functions of another licensed profession.

An unregulated athletic trainer may not legally perform the functions found in a state physical therapy practice act, regardless of the fact that the functions may be common to both professions and regardless of the fact that the functions fall within the domain of athletic training as published by the NATA board of certification.

Certification

Certification as a legislative regulatory act is separate from the NATA board of certification. In the state regulatory context, certification is less restrictive than licensure. Certification does not restrict the use of a title, such as athletic trainer, to certain individuals. However, it can restrict certain performance functions to only those practitioners who are regulated. State certification indicates to the discriminating public that one practitioner has expertise above and beyond that of another within the specific sphere of practice. A state certified practitioner has met higher standards of education, experience, or a combination of the two. Commonly, a state certified practitioner has also passed some form of a test given by the state itself. State certification is appropriate for those professions that pose less risk to public safety. Many allied health professions might be better regulated through certification as compared to licensure. At the time of this publication, seven states possess certification for athletic trainers (Table 3-2).

In contrast, the NATA certification examination is a validated and reliable national test of the knowledge and competency necessary to enter the practice of athletic training. Passing the NATA certification examination does not, in and of itself, grant a person a state certificate of regulation. Granting a certificate of regulation, whether it is a license or a certificate, is the prerogative of the state. Further confounding the confusion between state certification and NATA certification is the fact that regulatory agencies in nearly every state prefer the NATA certification examination as the test for knowledge and com-

---

Table 3-2
States that Certify Athletic Trainers

Kentucky	Pennsylvania
Louisiana	South Carolina
New Hampshire	Tennessee
New York	

petency of athletic training. Moreover, in many states, passing the NATA certification examination is the major criterion that grants a certificate of state regulation.

Registration

Registration is the least restrictive form of regulation. Registration is nominally seen as a listing of practitioners of a profession who have identified themselves to the state. However, registration does provide title protection for practitioners because no one can use the specified title unless the state grants its use. Normally, registration is granted if an appropriate fee is paid and certain educational criteria are met. Registration is often thought of as a revenue-generating mechanism for a state. At the present time, six states maintain registration (Table 3-3).

Exemption

Exemption also needs to be discussed. Exemption is the political process through which a state legislature recognizes that functions of an identified, though unregulated, profession duplicate those of a licensed profession. Without exemption, practitioners of the former profession would be in violation of the practice act of the latter profession. Exemption is not state regulation, per se, but it does provide legislative recognition of a particular profession. In most circumstances, exemption is mandated when the numbers of practitioners of a profession are too few to warrant the expense of regulation. Of course, exemption does not seem appropriate when practitioner numbers grow larger or when public demand for the "nonduplicated" services increase to the point of causing confusion between professions. Nor does exemption bode well as a basis for state supervision of a profession when the topic of reimbursement for services becomes noticeable. Table 3-4 represents a sample of states that have been provided exempt status in alternative practice acts.

Table 3-3
States that Register Athletic Trainers

Idaho	Missouri
Kansas	New Jersey
Minnesota	Oregon (voluntary)

Table 3-4
States that Exempt Athletic Trainers

Arizona (from physical therapy practice act)
Connecticut (from physician assistant practice act)
Colorado (from medical practice act)
Hawaii (from physical therapy practice act)

*The District of Columbia has judicial recognition of athletic training

Table 3-5
Sites of Practice of Athletic Training

Traditional Setting Only

Arizona	Nebraska	Pennsylvania
Colorado	New Hampshire	Rhode Island
Hawaii	New Jersey	South Carolina
Louisiana	North Dakota	Tennessee
Massachusetts	Oklahoma	

Clinical Setting Allowed

Alabama	Illinois	Mississippi
Arkansas	Indiana	New York
Delaware	Kentucky	Ohio
Idaho	Minnesota	

Setting Not Defined

Connecticut	Kansas	Oregon
Florida	Missouri	South Dakota
Georgia	New Mexico	Texas

Scope of Practice

The practice of athletic training is defined by the domains of athletic training as set forth by the board of certification of the NATA. Discussion of the scope of practice of athletic training is beyond the scope of this chapter. Suffice to say, however, that regulated athletic trainers must know what functions they can and cannot perform and stay within the confines of the regulation.

Athletic training practice parameters set by legislation generally fall within five areas:
1. Definition of athletic training or of athletic trainer
2. Site of practice restrictions
3. Modality use restrictions
4. Definition of athlete restrictions/physically active
5. Supervision of athletic trainers

Athletic trainers are usually defined as those who are engaged in athletic training and who are legally able to do so.[2] Subsequently, the definition of athletic training becomes important. In Maine, for example, athletic training is defined as "prevention, recognition, evaluation, management, treatment, disposition, and rehabilitation of athletic injuries as well as organization and administration of an athletic training program, to include education and counseling."[3] Each of these definitions is repeated in many of the regulatory acts in athletic training, with minor modifications. In essence, athletic trainers perform athletic training functions that are similar to those found in the language of the domains of athletic training from the NATA Board of Certification.

Site of practice restrictions are more pervasive. During the late 1970s and early to mid-1980s, many states passed athletic training practice acts that restricted athletic trainers to scholastic, collegiate, or professional sport training rooms. The growth spurt of sports medicine clinics was still on the horizon and the clinical role of athletic trainers was in the early stages. In that era, athletic trainers were happy to accept setting or site restrictions in order to get their bill through the objections of other allied health professions.

Realizing that the expanded role of clinical athletic trainers had forced the issue of site restrictions, those states that had that type of law in effect faced the unenviable situation of amending the athletic training practice act to allow clinical practice.

In opening up the act for amendment purposes, any law is available for any type of amendment from any other group with an interest in the act. Occasionally, amendments can be more restrictive than the original language.

In those states that restrict athletic training to the "traditional setting," athletic trainers who are employed in clinical settings are hired as physical therapy aides or physical therapist assistants (in those states that do not regulate physical therapist assistants) (Table 3-5). The problem for clinical athletic trainers lies in those states that have physical therapist assistant regulations and no athletic training regulations. The athletic trainer is then forced to work under the title of an aide. Aides are generally not allowed direct patient contact, unless the supervising physical therapist is willing to delegate specific patient duties to the athletic trainer under the aegis of the supervisor's license. Such conditions effectively prevent the non-athletic public from receiving the athletic training services that may be demanded.

Very few states limit the use of modalities in athletic training regulations. Delaware allows the athletic trainer to use modalities in the clinical setting. Alabama, Pennsylvania, South Dakota, and Colorado require a specific college-level course on modalities. Mississippi limits use of modalities to musculoskeletal injuries of the extremities only. Hawaii restricts the use of modality types to whirlpools and hot/cold pack application.

Limitation of the practice of athletic training can also occur from narrowly defining the term "athlete." Many states, particularly prior to the mid-1980s, defined an athlete as "an individual who participated in interscholastic, intercollegiate, professional or sanctioned amateur athletics." Providing services to "recreational" athletes was outside the parameters of athletic training, again despite the fact that those athletes were requesting the same type of service performed by the same type of regulated health care professional that treated the sanctioned athlete.

In the 1990s, the definitions showed a trend to include activities such as strength, agility, flexibility, range of motion, speed, and stamina in characterizing an athlete. Under this type of definition, athletic trainers were able to respond to the needs of the recreational and industrial athlete, and therefore, broaden the practice of athletic training.

The final area of restriction of the practice of athletic training is in supervision. Athletic trainers have long enjoyed a close working relationship with team physicians. Early definitions of athletic training included language that specified supervision by physicians. In all but four states (Maine, Florida, Arizona, Nebraska), physicians are designated as supervisors of athletic trainers. Physician supervisors are further defined as team and/or consulting physician in 14 states. Physician supervision in several states is actually extended over the practice of athletic training by the requirement that the physician review and agree to sign practice protocols that indicate what an athletic trainer may do in any given injury situation. Additional restrictions may be placed on athletic trainers to refer an athlete or patient that does not improve within a given amount of time back to the physician for re-evaluation. Nonphysician health care practitioners are also allowed to supervise athletic trainers in certain situations, generally in the clinical setting (Table 3-6).

Table 3-6

Non-Physician Supervision of Athletic Trainers

Physical Therapists (Clinical Setting Only)	**Chiropractors**	**Dentists**	**Physician Assistants**
Arizona	Delaware	Illinois	Iowa
Delaware	Illinois	Massachusetts	
Minnesota	Indiana	Ohio	
Mississippi	Ohio		
Ohio			

CHALLENGES TO REGULATION OF ATHLETIC TRAINING

Regulation of athletic training faces new demands other than those first envisioned in 1976. Regulation is now seen as a barrier to reducing costs of the health care delivery systems. Recent attempts by the federal government to revamp the health care industry underscore the need to control costs. Even as athletic trainers hear from third-party payers that professional regulation is critical to being reimbursed for services provided, there is a movement to reduce regulation. Reduction of regulation would allow for expanded spheres of practice for all professions, promote innovative health care programs, and encourage cost-effective and outcome-based health care protocols. The marketplace would drive the health care system. Professions would be allowed to venture into areas traditionally closed to them if the profession could prove through outcomes data reports that health care was both improved and less costly. Payers would become powerful as they demanded proof of success individually or industry-wide before reimbursing for services provided.

The consumer would need to be very discriminating in this type of system by always needing to pick a provider that could be reimbursed by a payer. Otherwise, the consumer would end up paying for services out of pocket.

Regulation is also seen as being closely linked to the education of practitioners. Regulatory scopes of practice should be drawn from the actual experiences of the practitioners and also should be reflected in the educational preparation of students. Clinically effective protocols would be reflected in both the educational preparation and in the scope of practice.[4]

In any respect, regulation cannot answer all of the questions that concern athletic trainers. Regulation cannot guarantee employment or reimbursement. Regulation cannot fulfill the need for acceptance as an allied health professional by other health professionals. These types of concerns are better relieved at the local or individual level. Regulation can and should, however, protect the public from unqualified practitioners.

Study Questions

1. Explain how the regulatory process has evolved with respect to athletic trainers.
2. Define licensure. What are the advantages and disadvantages of practicing athletic training in a state that recognizes licensure as a form of regulation?
3. Define certification as it relates to regulation. How does this differ from

the certification that is granted to athletic trainers following a passing score on the NATA certification examination?

4. What is the intent of registration as a form of regulation? Are there benefits for an athletic trainer practicing in a state that recognizes registration as a form of regulation?

5. How is exemption important with respect to the practice of athletic training?

6. List the common parameters that are typically identified when defining a scope of practice for athletic trainers. Can you think of any other parameters that may be beneficial to protect the practice of athletic training?

7. What is the scope of practice in the state where you currently practice? How does this affect what you are legally capable of performing as compared to the domains of athletic training?

References

1. Proceedings of the National Athletic Trainers' Association. Chicago, March 17, 1976.
2. Minnesota Athletic Trainers' Act. Minnesota Chapter Law 232, Section 148.7801-148.7815;1993.
3. Maine Athletic Training Licensure Act. MRSA Chapter 127-A, Sections 14351-14359;1995.
4. U.S. Department of Health and Human Services. Reports of the National Commission on Allied Health. Rockville, Md;1995.

Suggested Readings

Alabama Athletic Training Licensure Act. Act #93-617, 1993.

State of Arkansas 1995 AR H.B. 2074.

Arizona Revised Statutes. Title 32, Chapter 19, Article 2, A.R.S. @ 32-2021 (1991).

California Code of Regulations. Title 5, Division 1, Chapter 6, Subchapter 2, Article 5, 5 CCR 5593 (1995).

State of Colorado. 1995 CO H.B. 1002.

Connecticut General Statute @ 19a-16a, Title 19a, Chapter 368a (1990).

Delaware Practice Act. 24 Del., C., Chapter 26 (1993).

Delaware State Examining Board of Physical Therapy Rules & Regulations. Chapter 26 (1993).

State of Florida. 1995 FL H.B. 2413.

Rules of Georgia Board of Athletic Trainers. Chapter 53-1 - 53-9 (1989).

Hawaii Code Annotated. Division 2, Title 25, Chapter 461J, HRS @ 461J-3 (1991).

Idado Code, General Laws. Title 54, Chapter 39, Idaho Code @ 54-3913 (1991).

State of Illinois. 1995 IL H.B. 481.

Indiana Administrative Code. Title 898, Article 1, Rule 1, 898 IAC 1-1-1 (1995).

Code of Iowa. Title IV, Subtitle 3, Chapter 152D, Iowa Code @ 152D.1 (1995).

State of Kansas. 1995 KS S.B. 57.

Kentucky Revised Statutes Annotated. Title XXVI, Chapter 311, Subchapter: Athletic Trainers, KRS Ann. @ 311.900 (1991).

State of Louisiana. S.B. 714 (1995).

State of Maine. H.B. 699 (1995).

The Commonwealth of Massachusetts Regulation Filing and Publication. 259 CMR 1.00 - 5.00 (1994).

Minnesota Administrative Code. Chapter 3700, Minn. R. 3700.0435 (1994).

Mississippi Bill Tracking Statenet. 1992 MS S.B. 2475.

Revised Statutes of the State of Missouri. Section 334.700 R.S. Mo. (1990).

Revised Statutes of Nebraska. Chapter 71, Article 1, R.R.S. Neb. @ 71-1,240 (1990).

New Hampshire Revised Statutes Annotated. Title XXX, Chapter 326-G, RSA 326-G:1 (1994).

State of New Jersey. Division of Law and Public Safety, N.J.S.A. 45:9-37.35 (1984).

The State of New Mexico Statutes, Rules and Regulations. Athletic Trainers Practice Board, Article 14D, 61-14D-1 - 61-14D-9 (1994).

State of New York. Assembly Rule 3, Section 2, Article 167 (1991).

North Dakota Athletic Trainers Sct. Chapter 490, HB 1270 (1991).

North Dakota Century Code. Title 43, Chapter 43-39, N.D. Cent. Code @ 43-39-01 (1991).

Ohio Administrative Code. Chapter 3301-27, OAC Ann. 3301-27-02 (1994).

Oklahoma Athletic Trainers Act. Chapter 25, Title 59 O.S., Section 528 (1991).

Oregon Legislative Assembly. Chapter 744, S.B. 167 (1993).

Pennsylvania Administrative Code. Title 49, Part I, Subpart A, Chapter 40, Subchapter A, General Provisions 49 Pa. Code @ 40.5 (1995).

State of Rhode Island and Providence Plantation. Chapter 60 (1988).

Code Laws of South Carolina. Chapter 61, S.C. Code Regs. 61-96 (1993).

State of South Dakota. General Provisions, Chapter 20:63:01 (1993).

General Assembly of The State of Tennessee. Tennessee Code Annotated, Section 63-24-101 (1993).

Texas Administrative Code. TAC 313, Article 4512d (1995).

West Virginia Code annotated. Chapter 18A, Article 4, W. Va. Code @ 18A-4-16 (1995).

CHAPTER

4

The Health Care Delivery System

Marjorie J. Albohm, MS, ATC

OBJECTIVES

Upon completion of this chapter, the student will be able to accomplish the following:

1. Be familiar with the evolution of health care delivery systems

2. Understand the managed care health care delivery system, its components, and its various forms

3. Recognize the role of the athletic trainer as a health care provider in future health care delivery systems

The health care industry is in the process of undergoing the biggest change in history. The system of health care delivery, as we have known it, may never again be the same. The radical change that is underway will have a dramatic effect on health care providers, payers, and consumers of health care services.

Historically, Americans have enjoyed the freedom of choosing their health care providers, being appropriately treated, and being reimbursed partially or fully by health insurance for the services provided. Traditionally, that health insurance was paid for by the patient's employer. This payment system was known as a fee-for-service and the insurance policies providing coverage were called indemnity policies.

Skyrocketing health care costs have caused this traditional system to change dramatically. In 1992 the cost of health care in the United States was estimated at 838.5 billion dollars.[1] By the year 2000, the nation's annual health care cost is expected to reach nearly 1.7 trillion dollars annually.[2] The result of this is that employees will pay a higher percentage of their health insurance premium, or they may find themselves without any health insurance at all. Consumers, employers, and payers have begun demanding accessible, appropriate, cost effective, high quality health care. Traditional, fee-for-service indemnity coverage has become a system of the past.

Policy makers are debating the ultimate designs that health care should take in the future. Those involved in health care; including providers, payers, employers, state governments, and vendors have rapidly and aggressively altered their organization and business plan to meet the challenges of this rapidly changing system.[3] Although the final product is still unknown, some very clear health care organizational and delivery patterns are emerging, and will ultimately become the health care plans of the future.

MANAGED CARE

A major response to concerns of rising health care costs and to health care reform is managed care. Managed care is a system of health care that integrates the financing and delivery of health care services to participating individuals. Under this system, arrangements are made with selected providers to deliver comprehensive health care services. Standards for provider selection, formal ongoing evaluation of quality assurance and utilization, and a system of financial incentives to encourage member's use of providers are associated with the plan.[2] The overall goal of managed care is to control costs while maintaining quality.

Various methods are employed to oversee and control the care received, the amount paid to providers for services rendered, and the amount consumers pay for basic and supplemental care. Managed care combines the traditional roles of insurance companies (paying for health care) and health care providers (overseeing and delivering care).[2] In the traditional fee-for-service, specialty dominated, medical environment, there is no delivery system infrastructure to efficiently and economically manage health care.

Managed care is not a totally new concept. The existence of health maintenance organizations (HMOs), a major type of managed care program, can be traced back to the late 1920s. Well-known managed care organizations such as Group Health Cooperative of Puget Sound and The Kaiser Health Plan of California began in the mid-1940s and today represent some of the largest HMOs in the United States.

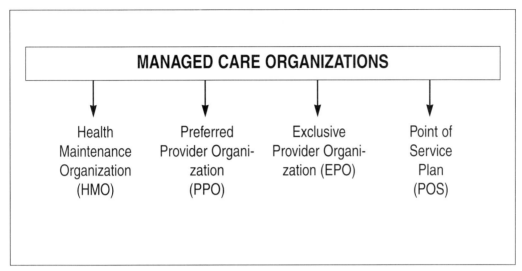

Figure 4-1. Types of managed care organizations.

The growth of managed care has been dramatic since the 1970s. A recent study report- ed that at the end of 1993, more than 44 million people belonged to 566 HMOs.[3] Experts believe that within this decade managed care will account for more than 80% of health insurance coverage in the United States.

Managed care plans designate a group of providers with whom members must consult. These providers are compensated by a predetermined rate. This may be either a salary or fixed amount and is based per program member, not for each service provided. Members, or their employers, pay a fixed monthly amount, but pay nothing or a small amount for each visit. Initial consultation with a primary care physician is required to determine the course of treatment and to make referrals to designated specialists, if needed.

Types of Managed Care Organizations

There are four major types of managed care organizations: 1) Health Maintenance Organizations (HMOs); 2) Preferred Provider Organizations (PPOs); 3) Exclusive Provider Organizations (EPOs); and 4) Point of Service Plans (POS) (Figure 4-1). Of these four, HMOs and PPOs seem to be the most common.

Although there are differences between each one of these plans, there exist some basic similarities. An established group of providers that members can access is central to each plan. A negotiated payment per member is provided rather than a traditional fee-for-service.

The differences between the plans are basically related to which providers are includ- ed in the network, which providers a member may consult, and provider accountability to the managed care organization for the services provided. Health care plans are usually categorized into one of these four models. Although in reality, specific plans may utilize some components of several models to formulate their organization.

An HMO is an organization of health care personnel and facilities that provides a defined range of health services to an enrolled population, for a fixed sum of money that is paid in advance, for a specified period of time.[4] The choice of providers is usually limit- ed to the HMO's network of physicians and hospitals.

The member pays a fixed annual premium, rather than a fee-for-service. The HMO is responsible for ensuring that the expenses involved in providing care will not exceed the premiums paid.

In a PPO, a third party (insurer, employer, administrator, or other sponsoring group) negotiates discounted rates for services directly with selected groups of providers.[2] Members may utilize providers outside of the network but increased copayments are required. Providers in a PPO are chosen on their qualifications and performance. They agree to a fee schedule and utilization managed procedures.

In an EPO, a group of providers contract with an insurer, employer, third-party administrator, or other sponsor. The provider agrees to the negotiated level of reimbursement. They agree to follow utilization review procedures and have patients admitted only to contracted hospitals. Unlike PPOs, the EPO provider can be prohibited from treating any patient not enrolled in the organization.[2] Members must seek services from participating providers in order to obtain reimbursement.

A POS plan is a mix between the HMO and PPO. In a POS plan, members receive care provided by network participating providers, but have the option of obtaining care outside the network.[2] HMOs and PPOs may offer POS plans to members as a way to expand member options. If a member receives care from a provider affiliated with an HMO or PPO, reimbursement is provided, but often with a higher copayment. If care is provided by a non-network provider, reimbursement may be significantly decreased. POS plans are usually more restrictive (similar to an HMO) for primary care and less restrictive (like a PPO) for specialty and ancillary care.

Components of Managed Care Organizations

All managed care plans share common components designed to deliver health care services to its members and to control costs.

Organized provider networks are central to most managed care programs. Members are encouraged or required to seek care from within the network. Networks allow the managed care organization to control utilization of services and therefore, cost of care. Providers in the network are compensated by the number of members enrolled or by salary, rather than by fee-for-service.

Utilization review is a specific process of managing health care services provided and the cost of those services. The process involves medical professionals outside the managed care organization reviewing the activities of the providers in the network, to evaluate the medical necessity and effectiveness of the treatments prescribed for specific conditions.[2] Some organizations utilize an internal utilization review program while others contract with independent firms.

Another way to control utilization is by reimbursing providers based on efficiency. Providers receive a salary or fixed payments based on the number of participants enrolled in the plan (known as capitation). Because a fee-for-service payment system is not utilized, excess and over-utilization is not encouraged. In fact, bonuses are often awarded for meeting established utilization goals.

Members of managed care organizations seeking care must often first consult a primary care physician for the establishment of a treatment plan, including the need for any subsequent referrals. This is referred to as "gatekeeping." The "gatekeepers" function is to reduce health care utilization and costs.

Incentives are often provided to members who only utilize the providers in their network. In some plans, reimbursement is provided only when network physicians are utilized. Other plans may allow out-of-network treatment, but require a high copayment.

Concerns about Managed Care

The most frequently expressed concerns regarding managed care are related to choice, quality, and cost savings. In America, citizens have always had "freedom of choice" in regard to their health care. Managed care plans generate many concerns regarding potential limitations on choice of provider, preference to see the same provider during the course of treatment, and access to specialists if uncommon conditions exist. In response to the choice issue, managed care organizations have broadened their provider networks and allowed members to access out-of-network providers (for additional fees). Specialist care is obtained through specific referral guidelines.

Determining standards for quality and monitoring and enforcing those standards is an ongoing concern throughout health care. Because provider incomes are tied to cost containment in managed care, a concern exists that providers may tend to underserve patients. Quality assurance systems designed to assess quality and evaluate performance have been instituted in most managed care organizations. Practice guidelines, developed by medical societies, have been developed and are utilized to improve quality and reduce practice variations.

Concern exists regarding access to specialty care through "gatekeeper" referrals. In a managed care system, financial incentives are provided to physicians for cost containment relevant to utilization of specialty consultations. This may result in inappropriately underutilizing specialty services. In addition, the background and experience level of the general practice physician serving as "gatekeeper" may not be sufficient enough to appropriately evaluate when specialty services may be needed. It is impossible to be thoroughly trained and extensively experienced in all of the specialty areas that are represented by individual patient complaints and disorders.

It is essential that primary care physicians, acting as "gatekeepers," promptly and accurately render diagnoses and, when necessary, recognize the need to refer patients to other specialists. That referral should be accomplished in a timely fashion so as not to jeopardize the resolution of the medical problem presented. A delay in the recognition of disorders and inappropriate follow-up treatment can certainly add to the patient's length of disability and functional limitation.

It has been difficult to accurately ascertain exact financial benefits of managed care simply because of its rapid evolution and the variations that exist in organizations. Theoretically, however, managed care should produce significant savings. Recent reports published by the Congressional Budget Office have indicated significant estimated and projected savings under managed care.[5]

Growth of Managed Care

Despite skepticism and criticism, managed care continues to grow and expand. Physicians are realizing that they must embrace managed care and become involved in managed care organizations in order to survive.

In some markets, physician specialists have reacted negatively to the advances of managed care organizations. Environments which may have dedicated their capital resources to high costs and specialized inpatient technology, have been forced to reshape their thinking and plans for the future.

Payers are taking the initiative to build, direct, and control managed care delivery systems in many cases. The large insurance carriers have concluded that they cannot depend on revenue generated from administering insurance functions alone. The payers, therefore, in markets in which managed care efforts of hospital systems and physician groups have been dormant, have aggressively created new health care delivery systems by building primary care facilities and contracting and employing primary care physicians.[6]

Government managed health care delivery systems such as Medicare and Medicaid are not immune to the issues of health care reform and the move to managed care. Managed care penetration has been significant in these systems. Many states have adopted some form of managed care to improve access to health care, ensure its quality, and manage costs. The use of managed care is evident in Medicaid, state employee benefit plans, and workers' compensation programs. It is projected that in the future the majority of participants in these government-sponsored health care plans will be enrolled in HMO models.

The development and implementation of a comprehensive, integrated system of health care delivery is occurring at a rapid pace throughout the United States. Provider networks and alliances are forming at all levels, with the goals of consolidating services, reducing costs, and improving efficiency in anticipation of a fully integrated managed care delivery system.

Managed Care and the Athletic Trainer

As health care progresses toward an organization of managed care, allied health professionals, specifically athletic trainers, must assess their position in a rapidly changing marketplace. Payers are demanding to know the value received for their dollar, and are in the process of continually comparing one provider to another. Providers must show value and objective documented benefits for dollars reimbursed. In reality, payers are looking for the lowest cost services available, maintaining and ensuring quality outcomes.

The health care services traditionally provided by athletic trainers have, in fact, been organized in a managed care fashion. Providing quality care in a cost efficient manner describes the role and function of the athletic trainer. Athletic trainers have long acted as physician extenders and case managers, providing a continuum of care ranging from prevention to restoration of normal function.

However, athletic trainers have not traditionally had an entrepreneurial approach in relation to promoting their skills and services to health plan developers. It is necessary for athletic trainers to validate their efficacy and efficiency and to promote their effectiveness to managed care organizations throughout the country.

The first step in accomplishing this is to participate in a scientifically designed outcomes data collection system. An objective outcomes data base is essential in demonstrating effectiveness and efficiency.

Outpatient rehabilitation services constitute a very small portion of the overall health care dollar and, therefore, often receive little attention from large payer groups. In order to capture that attention, athletic trainers must aggressively market their services and outcomes. In addition, they must further develop their relationships with family practice physicians, as well as musculoskeletal specialists. Reimbursement for athletic training services may be coupled with fees associated with physician provided services. Typically, large managed care organizations are not interested in negotiating with individual providers for individual services.

Athletic trainers must thoroughly educate themselves in the organization of managed care and must develop a state by state approach to managed care organizations to gain recognition and inclusion as providers in managed care networks.

Efforts directed at establishing communication with government managed health care delivery systems must be made and are already in progress in many states. Although athletic trainers do not typically become involved in providing health care to Medicare or Medicaid populations, many payers use these standards to determine reimbursable services and rates. Provider status can and should be sought from these entities.

Athletic trainers must establish their identity as recognized and accepted health care providers in the health care marketplace of the present and future.

The final shape of the health care delivery system in America has yet to be determined. It is hoped that the final product will be based on effectiveness, efficiency, quality, and consumer choice. Only then can it be said that health care has truly been reformed.

Study Questions

1. Discuss the evolution of health care reform.
2. Define and discuss the managed care health care delivery system and identify the central components of this system.
3. Identify and describe the four most common types of managed care organizations.
4. Identify and discuss the major criticisms of a managed care system.
5. Discuss the role of the athletic trainer in a managed care environment.

References

1. US Commerce Department. 1993 US Industrial Outlook, *Rocky Mountain News*. January 1993:4.
2. Harden SL. *What legislators need to know about managed care*. National Conference of State Legislatures; 1994:1–34.
3. Kenkel PJ. PPOs pursue new links with providers. *Modern Healthcare*. February 1992:42.
4. Medical Group Management Association. Managed care glossary of terms. MGMA, 104 Inverness Terrace East, Englewood, Colorado 80112-5306.
5. Wagner L. Universal HMO use offers savings. *Modern Healthcare*. September 1992:74.
6. Cochrand JD. Integrated delivery systems reposition for reform. *MGM Jour.* July/August:15–24.

Suggested Readings

Green K. *Managed Care: A health strategy for today and tomorrow*. Washington, DC: Health Insurance Association of America; 1993:53.

Modern Healthcare Journal. Modern Healthcare, Chicago, IL.

The Managed Care Health Care Handbook. Rockville, Md: Aspen; 1989

Employment in the Clinical Setting

Jeff G. Konin, MEd, ATC, MPT

OBJECTIVES

Upon completion of this chapter, the student will be able to accomplish the following:

1. Recognize the differences between employment in traditional and nontraditional settings

2. Identify factors considered essential to achieve job satisfaction

3. Recognize the signs and symptoms of burnout

4. Distinguish between desirable and undesirable employment opportunities

5. List important information that should be obtained prior to a potential job interview

Employment in the nontraditional athletic training setting has expanded recently to include physical therapy clinics, hospital-based clinics, industrial settings, and even personal fitness ventures that may entail multiple environments. Prior to this diversity, most athletic trainers could be found working in what are referred to as "traditional" settings. Traditional settings typically include high school, collegiate, and professional athletic environments.

An increasing number of certified athletic trainers as well as a growth in the educational preparation has led to the spread of athletic trainers into nontraditional settings. Initially, those athletic trainers who were employed in the nontraditional settings became accustomed to working typical 40-hour weeks that consisted of five 8-hour days, not including weekends. This was very appealing, because it was a very different time commitment than traditionally required. Athletic trainers employed in traditional settings can still expect to work long hours, including weekends, on a regular basis.

The employment expectations for nontraditional athletic trainers has greatly changed as a result of the clinical facilities' response to health care changes in the past 5–10 years. These changes have occurred primarily to 1) meet the needs of the increased demand for rehabilitation, 2) keep clinics abreast with competing regional facilities, and 3) satisfy insurance carriers who have tightened reimbursement policies.

The clinical, corporate, and industrial athletic trainer must be aware of the expectations to work in these types of settings. The purpose of this chapter is to prepare the athletic trainer who wishes to seek employment in a clinical setting with the information necessary to distinguish between desirable and undesirable potential employers in the nontraditional setting.

IMPORTANCE OF JOB STABILITY

It is well understood in any profession that a resumé that demonstrates multiple, short-stint employment terms brings forth many questions regarding the applicant's ability to maintain a position. In some cases, multiple job changes may be unplanned or uncontrollable, such as in family transfers. However, it usually represents a suspect employee.

It is not uncommon for people to be in a position in which their personality and skills do not match the conditions and expectations of an employment site. When this is the case, it becomes a difficult decision as to whether or not one should "stick it out" for hopes of future improvement, or to seek alternative employment opportunities.

Job stability is not only recognized by employers as a strength, but it also gives the employee an edge of confidence when working in an environment that he or she has become more comfortable with over a period of time. In a profession in which communication is not only important, but can possibly influence the success of rehabilitation, stability at one job will also benefit the athletes and patients.[1]

One of the first things that an athletic trainer can do to enhance job stability and desirability is to adequately and thoroughly acquire as much information about a potential employer as possible. Information may be gathered formally, e.g., obtaining documents that the employer has made public. Or it may be gathered informally via personal communication with peers, colleagues, and friends. Regardless of the method of collection, it is essential to ensure that the information is factual and not misleading. There are certain

Table 5-1
Turnover Factors and Management Actions
Encouraging Employee Retention

Factors Encouraging Turnover	Management Actions Encouraging Retention
Poorly defined position responsibilities	Clearly defined performance expectations
High-stress position	Management support to provide needed resources and remove obstacles that interfere with performance
Unchallenging work that does not utilize employee skills	Clearly define employee roles prior to employment
	Create clinical and management opportunities for advancement
	Design positions with performance expectations that match required skills
Unfair performance expectations	Involve employees in setting performance expectations
Lack of development opportunities	Provide frequent development opportunities that meet both organizational and employee development goals
Lack of recognition for work accomplishments	Provide recognition for good performance
Lack of opportunity to express work-related dissatisfaction	Provide formal mechanisms and encourage employees to express dissatisfaction
Low flexibility	Allow for flexible hours and working arrangements
Pay inequities	Provide employees with financial compensation that reflects market conditions
	Avoid internal pay inequities
Lack of advancement opportunities	Provide opportunities for clinical and management advancement whenever possible
Low levels of autonomy	Adopt a participation style of management that allows employees autonomy based on ability
Competitive environment	Competitive position content and context
Undesirable geographic location	Provide social support to new employees
	Recruit employees who are comfortable with the size and environment of the community

Reprinted with permission from Nosse LJ, Friberg DG. *Management Principles for Physical Therapists*. Baltimore, Md: Williams and Wilkins; 1992:90.

questions that may be asked in an attempt to seek appropriate information prior to employment, and this will be discussed later in the chapter. In addition, Nosse and Friberg have outlined certain factors that encourage employee turnover and retention (Table 5-1).

Job Satisfaction

Being satisfied with a job usually translates to a longer working relationship with a particular company or employer. For athletic trainers, many different factors exist that can lead to individual job satisfaction. In a questionnaire distributed at a Great Lakes Athletic Trainers' Association meeting, Halterman and Perkins showed that athletic trainers in clinical settings were actually more satisfied with their jobs when compared to those in other settings.[2] Further, Buxton et al identified and ranked motivational components of high school, university, and clinical athletic trainers in the state of Hawaii.[3] They found that those athletic trainers employed in the clinical setting presented with slightly different viewpoints as to what they consider important motivating factors. Overall, differences in motivational factors were found to exist in respective areas possibly due to the organizational structure of each setting.

IMPORTANCE OF WORK

It appears that athletic trainers in all settings are motivated by the perceived "importance of work."[3] Importance of work has been defined by Herzberg as an "intrinsic reward" because it seems to be associated with job satisfaction.[4] Herzberg believes when a person is satisfied that his or her work is perceived as being important, it can lead to increased productivity.[5]

Job Growth

The ability to grow as a professional is something for which most people strive. Increased responsibilities and occupational promotions fill a level of satisfaction that a person yearns to achieve through professional maturity.

On the contrary, a lack of change in responsibilities and a prolonged period of time in a single role may lead to frustration, boredom, and eventually burnout. All three are counterproductive to good health care delivery and can diminish the enthusiasm and willingness of an athletic trainer to provide optimal care.

One specific area that athletic trainers utilize to seek professional growth is that of continuing education. Typically, yearly organizational conferences are held to allow for the fulfillment of continuing education units, which may be required by the National Athletic Trainers' Association as well as those states whose licensure or certification are renewed only with proof of professional growth through continuing education. These conferences may include national, district, and state athletic training symposiums, and they serve to further educate athletic trainers with relevant advances in the field of athletic training. They also provide for an atmosphere in which networking with colleagues may take place.

Many other continuing educational opportunities are offered through private organizations, hospitals, and other health care professions. Athletic trainers who are employed in a clinical setting are typically allotted a fixed amount of dollars that may be applied toward continuing educational opportunities. The money may be used for course tuition, travel, lodging, and/or meals, depending on the individual facility's policy.

Benefits

Business administrators will attest that the cost of providing benefits to an employee are in the neighborhood of approximately one third of a person's salary. For example, it will cost an employer an additional 10,000 dollars to pay for benefits for an employee who earns 30,000 dollars per year.

Satisfactory employee benefits may be one of the single most important components of job satisfaction. Benefits may include, but are not limited to: insurance for health, life, dental, and vision; individual retirement accounts; and stock options. Many factors contribute to the decision-making process of determining whether or not an employer's benefit package is suitable. This decision must be made based on the current and future circumstances of the employee, and may take into account such issues as family matters, spousal employment benefits, and health status among others.

Salary

Often, a potential employee appears to be most concerned about the particular amount of revenue that he or she will earn. Unfortunately, the salary range that a job offers does not always represent a true correlation of the attractiveness of the position. It is not uncommon to come across positions with high range salaries because employers have had a difficult time retaining their employees. Likewise, some positions may have extremely low salaries because employers know they can attract many applicants based on their established reputation. A potential employee should never base the weight of his or her decision regarding employment on salary alone.

Salary ranges for athletic trainers may vary tremendously. These ranges may be influenced by the type of setting, the geographical location, the job responsibilities, and the credentials and experience of an athletic trainer, among other things.[6,7]

According to the "Placement Vacancy Notice" issued by the NATA and "Byline" (an athletic trainer registry in Michigan) in 1994, the average entry-level salary for a 12-month period for hospital- and clinic-based athletic trainers was $23,847, and $28,117 for those possessing a bachelor's and a master's degree, respectively.[8]

Achieving Work-Related Goals

Buxton's work demonstrated that athletic trainers believe that the opportunity to achieve work-related goals is essential to motivation.[3] It is important for athletic trainers to be given adequate periods of time and resources to accomplish work-related tasks. Being able to reach a goal is self-satisfying and can lead to professional employee and employer growth. On the contrary, unrealistic and unattainable goals can reduce morale and also lead to occupational burnout through perceived failure.

Communication

The ability to communicate with others in a pleasant, nonhostile environment may be the single most important component that a person should assess on a daily basis. Most people will spend nearly one third of their lives side-by-side with the people with whom they work. These interactions may include consultations, decision making, debating, and problem solving. The ability to get along with others cannot be over-emphasized in an environment where communication is essential for satisfactory outcomes.[9,10] Techniques to enhance communication skills are discussed in Chapter 12.

Job Security

Although it is rewarding for an employee to remain at one location to demonstrate job stability, it is comforting to know that an employer will also remain on solid working ground and thus provide for job security. With changes in health care, it is not surprising to find clinical facilities downsizing clinical staff positions or even changing ownership. Therefore, it is important for a person to understand the state of operations of his or her current employer as well as any future plans that may affect staff positions.

Working Environment

Working in a clinical setting may be a very different experience for those who have grown accustomed to spending their days in the training room. Treatment schedules, billing procedures, and the age, conditions, and goals of patient populations are just a few of the many differences that may exist between traditional and nontraditional settings. A recent graduate would greatly benefit from spending some time volunteering and observing the daily activities and operations of a facility prior to accepting employment in a nontraditional setting.

Job Flexibility

Many people aspire for the ideal position that allows them "job flexibility." Job flexibility means different things to different people, and may range from the ability to simply alter treatment schedules to the allowance of time off from work to attend continuing education workshops. Job flexibility may also include company policies on sick leave and arrangements for personal emergencies. Although flexibility is often determined by individual employers, it is typically more difficult to make unexpected changes or changes on short notice in smaller-sized departments.

ATHLETIC TRAINER ATTRITION

It is important to recognize that it is not only possible to become dissatisfied with an employer or employment setting, but also with the occupation of athletic training itself. There appears to be some correlation between the components of satisfactory employment and athletic training attrition. Capel has identified the following reasons for athletic trainers leaving the profession:[11]

1. Entering private practice as a physical therapist
2. Returning to school
3. Relocating
4. Salary too low
5. Having limited opportunities
6. Aquiring greater employment with another job
7. Teaching
8. Working long hours

Occupational Burnout

Occupational burnout is defined as "a syndrome of physical and emotional exhaustion involving the development of both a negative self-concept and a poor or negative attitude toward one's job."[12] The notion of occupational burnout has been widely published in the health arena.[13-21]

This is not a new concept to the profession of athletic training. However, it is always a concern and should be taken seriously. Many authors have looked at how burnout affects athletic trainers.[11,22-26] It is believed that burnout may be linked to stress, which is a physiological and emotional component often associated with the pressures of being an athletic trainer.

Capel has identified that burnout in the athletic training profession is generally lower than other "helping" professions.[25] Factors such as long hours, high role conflict, high role ambiguity, and large numbers of people needing treatment all contribute to potential environments for burnout.

In an attempt to reduce the possibility of burnout from occurring, it is essential to recognize the fundamental factors that lead to stressful situations and implement strategies to counteract these situations.

Establishing clear job descriptions can be utilized to decrease conceivable ambiguity.[25,27] In addition, programs that teach communication skills, conflict management skills, stress management, and organizational strategies may be beneficial in reducing or eliminating the factors contributing to burnout.

It is imperative to treat occupational burnout in its early stages because it can lead to many unwarranted situations. Manifestations may include physical changes in the form of headaches or ulcers, as well as other conditions such as anxiety and depression.[17] Ultimately, occupational burnout may lead to job attrition.[11,12] Most importantly, there is evidence that burnout can affect the quality of care delivered.[13]

EMPLOYMENT PREPARATION

Most of the reasons why athletic trainers remain at their respective positions as well as the reasons for why they leave positions have been discussed. Many times it is very difficult to uncover pertinent information in a timely fashion to enable a person to make an educated decision regarding the status of future employment.

When is it appropriate to ask questions of potential employers? Is there an appropriate way to phrase certain questions? Are there some questions that should not be asked? There is no definite answer to these questions, as each individual circumstance will require the job candidate to adapt to the situation at hand.

There are, however, some important questions that should be addressed by the candidate either prior to or at the time of an interview. At the very least, they should be addressed prior to the accepting of a position by the candidate. This list of questions is by no means inclusive of all of the information that a person might need to make an educated decision regarding future employment. Instead, it serves as a foundation on which to develop some essential facts about a potential employer.

1. What are my roles and responsibilities as outlined in the job description?
2. What expectations do you have for me as my employer?

3. How long have the current staff members been employed at this facility?
4. What measures do you take to promote staff interaction, communication, and morale?
5. What measures are taken to provide for job flexibility?
6. Is time allotted for professional growth?
7. What types of opportunities exist for continuing education and professional growth?
8. What is the chain of command, and how are my ideas and opinions received?
9. What type of support staff is available?
10. Can you explain the benefits package that is available? Are other employees satisfied with the current benefits? Are there any future plans to change?
11. Where does this facility/company plan to be in the future?
12. What is the current salary? Do opportunities exist that may provide for supplemental income?
13. Are employee evaluations or performance appraisals used to assess performance?

There are many areas that should be addressed prior to accepting a position. Preparation is the key. Collecting factual information on a position enables a person to make educated decisions. The process of recruiting an athletic trainer for employment involves the gathering of information from both parties, the employer and the potential employee. For a candidate to sell his or her services, he or she should make a strong effort to ensure that a facility not only sells itself, but that it is compatible with his or her expectations and desires.

SUMMARY

The roles and responsibilities for athletic trainers may be slightly different in traditional and nontraditional settings.

Employment in nontraditional athletic training settings may include physical therapy clinics, hospital-based clinics, industrial settings, and personal fitness training.

Job satisfaction is an essential component for job stability. Many factors contribute to job satisfaction, including a perception of the importance of work, opportunities for job growth, benefits, salary, the ability to achieve work-related goals, communication, job security, working environments, and job flexibility.

Athletic trainer attrition is a realistic concern and may be related to job dissatisfaction. Job dissatisfaction may lead to occupational burnout. Occupational burnout can manifest itself both physically and emotionally, and is deleterious to the delivery of optimal health care.

Preparation is the key to being adequately and factually informed prior to the acceptance of a job. Athletic trainers should be prepared to ask questions and gather facts about potential employment opportunities.

Study Questions

1. Discuss the differences between working in traditional and nontraditional athletic training settings.
2. Explain the importance of job stability.
3. List the components that may determine job satisfaction, and explain the importance of each.

4. Identify reasons for athletic trainer attrition.

5. What is occupational burnout, and how can it manifest itself?

6. What are some early signs of occupational burnout?

7. What specific steps can one take to prevent occupational burnout in the athletic training profession?

8. Prepare a mock job interview. What questions would you ask of a potential employer? If you were the employer, what questions would you have for an athletic training job candidate?

References

1. Fisher AC, Scriber KC, Matheny ML, Alderman MH, Bitting LA. Enhancing Athletic Injury Rehabilitation Adherence. *J Ath Train*. 1993;28:312-318.

2. Halterman AR, Perkins SA. Job satisfaction among certified athletic trainers. *J Ath Train*. 1995;S-23. Abstract.

3. Buxton BP, Lankford SV, Gieck JH. Motivational congruency and discrepancy of Hawaiian athletic trainers. *J Ath Train*. 1992;27:326–333.

4. Herzberg F. *The Motivation to Work*. New York, NY: J Wiley & Sons; 1959.

5. Herzberg F. One more time: How do you motivate employees? *Harvard Business Review*. Sept–Oct, 1987;65:118.

6. Mangus BC, Golden G, Tandy R, Koloskie J. Employment characteristics of collegiate athletic trainers in the western United States. *J Ath Train*. 1992;27:158. Abstract.

7. Moss CL. Entry-level salaries for athletic trainers. *J Ath Train*. 1992;27:158. Abstract.

8. Moss CR. 1994 Entry-level athletic training salaries. *J Ath Train*. 1995;s-13. Abstract.

9. Davies GJ. The need for critical thinking in rehabilitation. *J Sport Rehab*. 1995;4:1-22.

10. Fisher AC, Hoisington LL. Injured athlete's attitudes and judgments toward rehabilitation adherence. *J Ath Train*. 1993;28:48-54.

11. Capel SA. Attrition of athletic trainers. *J Ath Train*. 1990;25:34-39.

12. Donohoe E, Nawawl A, Wilker L, Schindler T, Jette DU. Factors associated with burnout of physical therapists in Massachusetts rehabilitation hospitals. *Phys Ther*. 1993;73:11, 750-756.

13. Deckard GJ, Present R. Impact of role stress on physical therapists emotional and physical well-being. *Phys Ther*. 1989;69:713-718.

14. Freudenberger HJ. The staff burnout syndrome in alternative institutions. *Psychotherapy Theory Research Practice*. 1975;12:73-82.

15. Maslach C. *Burnout: The Cost of Caring*. New York, NY: Prentice Hall; 1982.

16. Maslach C, Jackson S. Burnout in health professions: A social psychological analysis. In: Sanders G, Sul J, eds. *Social Psychology of Health and Illness*. Hillsdale, NJ: Lawrence Erlbaum Associates; 1982.

17. Patrick PKS. Professional roles at risk for burnout. *Family Community Health*. 1984;6:25-31.

18. Pines A, Maslach C. Characteristics of staff burnout in mental health settings. *Hosp Community Psychiatry*. 1978;29:233-237.

19. Schuster ND, Nelson DL, Quisling C. Burnout among physical therapists. *Phys Ther*. 1984;64:299-303.

20. Stubbs D, Rooks C. The stress, social support and burnout of critical care nurses: The results of research. *Heart Lung*. 1985;14:31-39.

21. Wolfe GA. Burnout of therapists: Inevitable or preventable? *Phys Ther*. 1981;61:1046-1050.

22. Gieck J. Stress management and the athletic trainer. *J Ath Train*. 1984;19:155-119.

23. Gieck J, Brown R, Shank R. The burnout syndrome among athletic trainers. *J Ath Train*. 1982;17:36-40.

24. Cambell D, Miller M, Robinson W. The prevalence of burnout among athletic trainers. *J Ath Train*. 1985;10:110-113.

25. Capel SA. Psychological and organizational factors related to burnout in athletic trainers. *J Ath Train*. 1986;21:322-327.

26. Vergamini G. *Professional burnout: Implications for athletic training*. 1981;16:197-198.

27. Ray RR. Performance evaluation in athletic training: Perceptions of athletic trainers and their supervisors. *J Ath Train*. 1991;26:148.

Suggested Readings

Buxton BP, Lankford SV, Noda LS. Motivational congruency and discrepancy between certified athletic trainers and noncertified student athletic trainers in the state of Hawaii. *J Ath Train*. 1992;27:320-324.

Duncan KM, Wright KE. A national survey of athletic trainer roles and responsibilities in the allied clinical setting. *J Ath Train*. 1992;27:311-316.

Okerlund VW, Jackson PB, Parsons RJ. Factors affecting recruitment of physical therapy personnel in Utah. *Phys Ther*. 1984;74:177-184.

Ray RR. Athletic trainer performance: Standards for development of the evaluation systems. *J Ath Train*. 1991;26:225-226.

Weidner TG. Sports medicine centers: Aspects of their operation and approaches to sports medicine care. *J Ath Train*. 1988;23:22-26.

Planning a New Athletic Therapy Facility

Julie Moyer Knowles, EdD, ATC, PT

OBJECTIVES

Upon completion of this chapter, the student will be able to accomplish the following:

1. Identify the 16 influencing considerations when planning a new athletic therapy facility

2. Describe the 16 influencing considerations when planning a new athletic therapy facility

3. Prioritize the 16 influencing considerations when planning a new athletic therapy facility

4. Form a time line involving the 16 preliminary considerations, starting at 18 months prior to opening and ending the day the facility opens

A lot of thought and effort must occur prior to building an athletic therapy practice. Before the doors of the facility ever open, there are at least 16 preliminary considerations that must be addressed. It is the purpose of this chapter to present each of these 16 considerations and discuss the implications for an athletic therapy facility.

LOCATION

There are several preliminary functions that need to occur before beginning a new athletic therapy facility. One of the first is identifying the location of the facility. Where will the facility be located? Will the zoning allow for the facility? Who are the referring doctors in that area? Are any of the referring doctors known or familiar, or has a relationship been established in the past with these physicians so that the athletic trainer will be more inclined to get their referrals in the future? What different businesses and schools are there in the area that are marketable for their sports medicine business or industrial rehabilitation on-site assessment business? Are there any other similar therapy practices that may directly or indirectly compete with the new business?

NAME

Besides location, another important preliminary decision athletic trainers need to make concerns the name of the business. Will the name be location specific? Will it be subspecialty specific? Will the athletic trainer's name be used? There are pluses and minuses to each. If the location is specifically defined, people will have a general idea where the business is located without having to define the location in the marketing material. However, the negative factor to having a location-specific name is that in the event of future growth, it may be a disadvantage to have a name-specific site. For example, a company called Washington, DC Athletic Therapy will be fine if it stays in Washington, DC. However, if it expands to Virginia, it may be confusing to call the second location Washington, DC Athletic Therapy.

There are pluses and minuses to subspecialty-specific names as well. Using Washington, DC Athletic Therapy as an example, some clients may not come to the facility because they feel the clinic only provides athletic therapy services. Obviously, an athletic trainer will have more emphasis in sports medicine, but may also want to treat a lot of non-sports-related injuries. By labeling the business in this manner, people with athletic injuries may tend to migrate toward the facility but those with other types of injuries may tend to stay away from the facility. An athletic trainer using his or her own name to name a business, will indeed help with personal marketing. It is very good for an athletic trainer to have his or her specific name associated with his or her specific practice so that doctors can identify the practice with the trainer. However, the downfall of solely naming the business after the trainer's name is that for a business to be successful, it requires the cooperative effort of all staff members. By solely naming it after the trainer's name, it may not give the recognition to other staff members, which they may indeed deserve. A compromise of this could be, for example, John Smith's Washington DC Athletic Therapy, Inc, where the reserved legal name is actually Washington, DC Athletic Therapy, Inc, but "John Smith" is before it on the marketing material to help identify the trainer with the corporation.

Once the facility's name is decided, the name will need to be protected. Nonincorporated businesses can reserve and protect their name by registering it with the prothonotary's office (most states) in each of the counties it will be operating. There is usually a minimal cost (approximately $15 for each county—a one-time fee) to do this. Any business that is incorporated is automatically registered and protected. The standardized forms for reserving other business names will include the business name, names of all its officers, the type of business structure, and the date it was formed. It also needs to be notarized and sent to a county public building, courthouse, or a county courthouse. In addition, most banks require that the athletic trainer/owner have his or her name registered to open up a business account. Failure to do this could result in a $500 fine.

STRUCTURE

The first thing to do in planning an athletic therapy facility is to determine the business structure. There are several different options. First, there is the *sole proprietorship*. This is the simplest form of business organization in which the entire business is owned by one individual. The advantage of sole proprietorship it that there is less paper work; however, all business operations are entirely tied into the owner's personal status including tax return status, and the owner is personally liable for actions incurred by the business. The second option is the *partnership,* in which two or more people under a contractual agreement are co-owners of the company. With this type of an arrangement there is unlimited liability for the partners, and again the income or loss is reflected on the partners' personal tax returns at the individual tax rate. The third, and most popular, business structure is a *corporation*.

Corporations involve ownership divided into shares of stock. The advantage of corporations is that they have perpetual life and the principal stock owners of the corporation face only a limited liability. That is, the corporation acts as a person in itself and there is less of a personal liability by the active clinician and the clinician's personal assets. There are three types of corporations that are used generally: 1) S corporation, 2) C corporation, and 3) limited liability corporation (LLC). The *S corporation* allows for the personal profits or losses of the corporation to be reflected on the individual stockholder's personal income tax, thereby being taxed at his or her personal income tax rate proportional to the amount of stock that he or she owns. Another advantage of an S corporation is the ease in selling the business compared with a C corporation. (It is advantageous for new businesses to start up as a sub-chapter S corporation because most new businesses will for the first 2–5 years show a loss that could directly be reflected on the stockholder's own personal tax return.) A *C corporation* does not filter the profits or losses to the individual directly. The corporation itself pays taxes at a corporate tax rate. An *LLC* is a corporation in which stockholders may actually be other corporations, not just individuals as with S corporations and C corporations. Prospective owners should contact the secretary of State Division of Corporations in their own state to receive forms and assistance for forming a corporation and to receive the certificate of incorporation. Corporations must have an office located in the state they are registered (not a post office box), must submit an annual report, pay franchise tax, maintain a registered agent (in many cases this is a lawyer), and pay corporate income tax if operating in the state.

There are several people who can help in selecting what type of business structure would be best for the needs of the facility. Common contacts are the U.S., state, or county Chamber of Commerce, a university's Small Business Developmental Center, the U.S. Small Business Administration (SBA), the Service Corps of Retired Executives (SCORE), and a personal lawyer and/or accountant.

TAXES AND LICENSES

The next decisions that have to be made in the preliminary planning of an athletic therapy practice involve taxes and licenses. If the practice is set up as a sole proprietorship or partnership, the income or loss of these should be reflected on 1) individual personal income tax, and 2) a partnership tax return. With a partnership tax return, any partnership having a resident partner, or any other income derived within the state, must file a return. The partnership itself will not be taxed, but each partner will be liable for state personal income tax on his or her share of partnership income. Information on sole proprietorship, partnership, or corporate income tax can also be obtained from the Division of Revenue.

Any domestic corporation must file an annual Franchise Tax unless specifically exempt by law. The initial cost is based on a company's authorized capital stock, either par value stock or non-par value stock. All domestic corporations have to file their annual Franchise Tax report of corporations before March 1 of each year. A minimum annual filing fee (about $20) and a Franchise Tax of not less than $30 or more than $150,000 must be submitted (as computed by the lessor amount). Information on the Franchise Tax can be obtained from the secretary of State Division of Corporations. The actual corporate income tax is computed on a corporation's taxable income, apportioned and allocated to the state at the specific tax rate (e.g., Delaware is 8.7%). An S corporation is required to make personal income tax payments to the state on behalf of its nonresident stockholders, so that the nonresidents are treated in the same manner as resident stockholders.

Some of the filing requirements of taxes by the company include an employer's identification number, federal income tax, federal employment tax, social security, U.S. immigration and naturalization, unemployment insurance, workers' compensation, state withholding, and job training tax. Applying for an employer's identification number should be one of the first steps when starting a new business. Form SS-4 must be filed, which can be obtained from the local IRS office at no cost, or 1-800-829-3676 can be called to receive a federal ID number to be used for all business transactions with the new business. The federal income tax withholdings are wages that the employer must withhold based on the employee's gross income, marital status, pay frequency, and withholding allowances as claimed on the W-4 form. Under the FUTA Act (Federal Unemployment Tax Act), employers are liable for federal unemployment taxes that are deposited quarterly on an IRS Form 940. Returns are filed annually and are due by January 31 of the following year. Social Security taxes were mandated by FICA (Federal Insurance Contribution Act), so that income for retired persons who have worked for a period of time before retirement may receive Social Security income. Both the employees and the employers pay FICA taxes on wages up to $60,000. Information is reported on Form 941.

The state withholding income tax system requires employers to register with the State

Division of Revenue, use their Federal ID number, and withhold an appropriate tax from employee compensation. The employer is responsible for supplying each employee with a statement showing the total wages earned and the amount of taxes withheld each year before January 31. The Job Training Tax, which was enacted through the Blue Collar Jobs Act of 1984, institutes a state assessment (about 1%) on wages paid by employers that are subject to State Unemployment Insurance taxes. The tax is collected through the state's Division of Unemployment Insurance. Another tax that may or may not need to be paid in addition to the aforementioned taxes is the Realty Transfer Tax, which in Delaware is a 2% state tax imposed on real estate transactions. Also, a person who may give you monies (in excess of $10,000 per donee per year) to help you start up the business may be responsible for a gift tax.

Employers must also complete Form I-9 within 3 business days of hiring a new employee, except if a person is self-employed. The I-9 Form is the U.S. Immigration and Naturalization form that ensures that illegal aliens are not being used as employees. All employers must also file Form UC1 and are liable for unemployment insurance taxes if they pay wages of $1,500 or more during any calendar year or employ one person more than 20 days during a calendar year. The unemployment insurance program contact person is at the Department of Labor, Division of Unemployment Insurance. All employers are also subject to their states' workers' compensation law that protects employers from employee liability for work-related injury or disease. Information can be obtained through the Industrial Accident Board, Division of Industrial Affairs.

Although the taxes seem overwhelming, there are some tax incentives in various states. If an employer qualifies, there are some areas that offer reduction in property taxes for economic development, some qualifying firms can receive a gross receipts tax reduction, and there may be a corporate income tax credit for qualified firms. There are some tax credits given for minority controlled firms, including majority owned female businesses, and tax credits for hiring individuals with physical or mental impairments.

In addition to taxes, a basic Business License must be obtained. An occupational license costs about $75 annually and $25 for each branch or additional business location, plus an approximate .4% fee on the taxable gross receipts in excess of $15,000 per month. This means that an annual fee is paid for having a license, and another fee is paid based on gross receipts (gross receipts tax) that are obtained each month in excess of $15,000 in some states, regardless of whether a profit or loss was incurred during that month. Licenses for a business can be obtained at any Division of Revenue office. The second type of license that an athletic trainer/owner must secure is a license to practice. Many states require that a licensed (permanent, not temporary) health care practitioner is present when patients are being treated.

FINANCIAL ASSISTANCE

Although many small businesses are established without financial assistance from outside investors or lenders, many people get started by going to banks or government agencies and requesting loans. Even if a company does not own property, it may be able to get a loan if it can show that there is an ability to repay the borrowed funds from future profits. One of the key agencies that helps with loans and financing is a State Development

Office and the Small Business Development Center. They host a number of small business seminars in coordination with area banks. The banking community is also very good at helping with financing and also integrating personal financing and loans with different government agencies, therefore it is essential to contact a good banker. When going to a bank for a small business loan, the bank will want to know background information including a client's ability to repay the loan, commitment to the project, any financial projects for at least 3 years, business experience, the type of collateral such as a house or other personal investments that a client may have, financial resources, and the client's general background. Many times a business plan must be presented, which explains how the client perceives his or her future business operations including profits and losses. This plan helps the bank determine the business's ability to repay the loan.

The bank may also require a co-signature on the loan if the client only has limited collateral. The lender must be convinced of the client's trustworthiness. Sometimes clinical owners are interested in establishing a line of credit, in which a loan can be given up to a certain amount of money over a period of time. There are a number of government agencies that also help with business plans and loans. The SBA guarantees loans with small companies agreeing to ensure up to 90% of the loans up to $155,000; and 85% of the loans greater than $150,000. SBA also offers non-monetary assistance in the form of advice through SCORE. It is also essential that the clinical owner have a detailed written business plan when contacting the bank.

LEGAL ADVICE

It is essential that good quality legal advice be obtained when starting a new business. An attorney can assist the clinical entrepreneur in many aspects of establishing a new business, including helping to incorporate the business, registering the name, assisting with the financial questions, and preparing contracts for other employees. A caution is the cost of legal advice.

RISK MANAGEMENT

Risk management is a plan that the clinical owner can take in order to minimize potential loss. Careful purchase of insurance along with sound management, evaluation of current and potential problems, and careful decision-making can help protect the individual and his or her business. The first step in risk management is defining the goals of the risk management program. The goals of the company include producing profits, maximizing profits through growth, and offering goods and services to customers while meeting legal and community obligations. After goals are selected, a policy statement should be formulated to establish the goals and community acceptance. Next, a list of all the risks that can cause loss to your business should be made. These include economic speculative risks (e.g., future national health care plans), personal risks involving the owner or employees (e.g., benefit liabilities), liability risks (e.g., malpractice), fidelity and surety risks (e.g., employee dishonesty and crime), property risks (e.g., equipment failure), statutory legal liability risks in which the company for some reason does not comply with federal statutes (e.g., noncompliance to Medicare guidelines), and net income risks in which the amount of income that is expected to cover costs is not produced. Finally, each risk must be analyzed and looked at for the potential of the risk occurring, the consequences, and what can be done to eliminate these hazards. Insurance policies can reduce these possible risks.

INSURANCE

Before buying insurance, the clinical owner needs to evaluate and investigate different insurance agents. Selecting a proper insurance broker/agent is critical in establishing a new business. The clinical owner needs to obtain references from different business professionals such as the bank, attorney, or accountant. Because most owners do not want to expose themselves to unnecessary liability, some insurance, such as workmen's compensation, is required by law, but other types of insurance are not required, yet are strongly suggested. Insurance policies that a clinical owner may need to evaluate include liability insurance, property insurance, workers' compensation insurance, automobile insurance, malpractice insurance, and home-based business insurance. *Liability insurance* covers the business from financial loss as a result of a business' negligence. This can include acts by the owner or the employees or even general business conditions. Liability insurance is not required but it is strongly suggested. *Property insurance* provides protection from damage or loss of property from fire, theft, employee dishonesty, and explosion. Rates depend on varying factors (e.g., whether the facility has a sprinkler system). Again, property insurance is not required but it is strongly suggested. *Workers' compensation insurance* is mandatory by law. This type of insurance protects the employer from liability for work-related accidents or diseases. Any authorized broker can provide workmen's compensation insurance and many times it is included in what is known as an umbrella policy. Umbrella policies cover several insurance needs all under one umbrella and it is a common form of policy for small new businesses. Workmen's compensation insurance information can be obtained from the Industrial Accident Board, Division of Industrial Affairs. *Automobile insurance* covers property and liability for any vehicles that are used during business hours. This does not have to cover the insurance from company-owned automobiles only. It may also cover possible accidents that are incurred; e.g, while an employee drives to the hardware store on company time. Automobile insurance can be obtained as an individual policy or may be part of another policy. For example, McGinnis & Associates, a common malpractice insurer, has a subsection that will allow for automobile insurance as well. In addition, McGinnis & Associates provides malpractice insurance for the employer and his or her employees. *Malpractice insurance* is essential, not only for the company and the employees in general, but it is also highly recommended for the individual to get on his or her own. If any part of a business is being done outside of the clinic, additional insurance will be needed to cover business assets and liabilities at home. Some clinicians have an office in the home and keep all business records there instead of in the clinic. *Home-based business insurance* can be obtained on a homeowner's insurance policy or through the business.

Health insurance needs to be evaluated for everyone. *Health insurance* is just one aspect of any entire employee benefit plan that should be established prior to the opening of the business. There are several different options in providing health insurance for employees: 1) the employer pays for the entire premium, 2) the premium is split, or 3) the employee is solely responsible. Providing health care insurance for small companies is very expensive. Therefore, one suggestion is for a small company to join a larger organization such as the Chamber of Commerce, where it can get reduced group rates for health care insurance. Other areas to be considered when thinking about health insurance are the deductible (the lower the deductible, the more costly the premium), the co-insurance, whether there will be major medical protection where there is a maximum out-of-pocket yearly cost for the co-insurance for the individual, and whether the health insurance will also be tied in with any other special plans (e.g., dental insurance, vision coverage, prescription cards). In addition, a clinical owner needs to evaluate whether the clinic needs a traditional health care plan or a health maintenance type of managed care plan. There are HMOs, PPOs, and many other plans out there to be evaluated for small groups.

A clinical owner must also think about other benefits, other than health care benefits, that he or she can offer his or her employees. This may include a life insurance policy, whether or not spouses and dependent children will be included, and a vacation policy, holidays, sick days, and personal days. A very general estimate is that it costs an employer approximately 20%–35% of the employee's gross salary for benefits. One recommendation for a clinical owner is to borrow a printed employee handbook from another facility and modify it for his or her particular facility. This will cut down on a lot of time and planning. An employee plan should be established prior to the start of a business if more than one person besides the owner will be employed by the facility.

BANK ACCOUNT

Once a tax ID number and an address and name of the corporation have been established, it is time to open a bank account. To open a bank account, a clinical owner needs the three items mentioned above, and a business license. If the facility is a corporation, a corporate seal is needed. This is obtained in the corporate kit, which a lawyer should have established. The clinical owner will need to fill out several forms including corporation resolution forms stating who can sign and withdraw money from the account. On this form, it must list whom the different officers of the corporation are, if incorporated. The form must be signed by the secretary of the corporation and a minimum fee in most cases of $50 must be deposited to open up the account. When the clinical owner starts a corporation, he or she can be listed as the president, vice president, secretary, and treasurer. If someone else becomes involved, it is wise for the clinical owner to keep him- or herself as the president and secretary because most of the important legal documents have to be signed by the president and secretary, and usually a second signature is not required. Checks can be used from the bank or can be purchased through a private supplier. Health Care Financing Administration (HCFA) billing forms also can be purchased from a private supplier.

SUPPLIES

Besides business checks and ledger systems, there are also many other supplies that are needed for the business office and clinic. Such supplies include pens, pencils, computers, typewriter, copier, fax machine, dictation equipment, files, progress sheets, exercise sheets, evaluation sheets, letterhead, business cards, telephones, some kind of music apparatus, lotion, towels, gowns, goniometers, and medical and taping supplies.

EQUIPMENT

In addition to supplies, equipment is needed also. Equipment includes things such as treatment tables (this will depend upon the amount of treatment rooms the facility will have), modalitic equipment, traction machines, exercise equipment, washers and dryers, whirlpools, whirlpool seats, ice machines, and hydroculators. It is suggested that when initially starting a business, machines that are the most versatile are purchased, that is, instead of buying one ultrasound and one electrical stimulator machine, you may want to buy an ultrasound/stim combination. Also, in terms of exercise equipment, it is suggested again that a machine that is highly versatile is purchased, such as a pulley machine that can be used by the arms or the legs, a bike ergometer that could either be used for biking one legged or two legged or as an arm ergometer, and some form of step machine that could be used for closed chain upper extremity or lower extremity exercises. Initially, large investments should not be made in equipment such as isokinetic testing until the referrals are determined and the types of service that physicians are seeking is investigated.

Other large equipment that may be worth investing in include a computer system and billing software package. Unless the bills go out in a prompt manner, cash flow will not be there and future bills will not be paid. One word of caution regarding billing and software packages: many software packages have been designed for physician's offices. For example, in a primary care physician's office, a person may see that physician once or twice a year and be billed for that one service received that day. In an athletic therapy practice, however, a person may see a trainer 12 or 15 days in a row and never again for the rest of his or her life. To have a billing software package that only prints out one service per page would then mean that there will be 12–15 pages of bills for the time the trainer saw the patient. This is very costly and not appropriate for athletic therapy. Therefore, when searching out a billing package, the clinical owner should make sure it is compatible to the hardware and visa versa, and that it can be adapted to the facility's needs. It is also wise to get the source code so that any future changes may be done by an independent consultant. Another decision to make with computers is what type of system to use (e.g., UNIX, DOS). Choosing a system is dependent upon how many different functions need to tie-in to the single computer. A computer should be purchased for the facility's current needs with the ability to adapt it for future needs. First-time business owners should not buy large, expensive, complicated computers thinking that they may need the strength years from now. Costs of computers and software change constantly, and upgrading software and hardware is inevitable; therefore, a clinical owner should buy for today but allow expansion for tomorrow. Also to be evaluated in equipment and supplies are salespersons for things such as braces, TENS units, and miscellaneous equipment. A good salesperson can really help direct a clinical owner in purchasing some equipment that may not be a big name brand but may be just as effective and a lot more cost-efficient. Many sales people will, on consignment, leave electrical units at the new facility, which may be used on clients there or be signed out for clients to use at home. This can really help a new clinic facility in that it may not need to purchase this equipment itself.

UTILITIES/LEASE

Before a new facility can start up, utility companies have to be notified of the start of business for the following services: electric, water, phone, and any other necessary utilities. Also, a lease for the building needs to be evaluated by a lawyer, or if the facility was purchased, all proper paper work should be filed by the accountant and lawyer. (Purchasing a building is not initially recommended.)

ADVERTISING

In order for a business to begin a full day of work on the first day, it must be advertised. A majority of the referrals that a clinic will get for athletic therapy are through physicians. It is essential that clinical owners meet with local physicians, introducing themselves and their business and providing materials, including a brochure listing their services and hours of operation, business cards, and prescription pads. Anyone who meets with a physician should be prepared to wait an hour to only see him or her for 30 seconds. This may seem like a waste of time initially, but patience and actually meeting with the physician will make it worthwhile in the long run. It is good marketing to take advertising paraphernalia (e.g., T-shirts, water bottles, and pens with the company logo) to the physician when visiting. It is possible to spend 10% of the facility's total expenses in the first year on advertising.

A new facility can advertise with youth groups, businessmen, coaches, and schools. Again, the various advertising paraphernalia, such as free T-shirts and water bottles, will definitely help a new business. The yellow pages in the phone book, although they may initially seem to be a good form of advertising, may be overly expensive for a new company. For example, an advertisement approximately 36½" x 4" in the yellow pages may cost $500 per month. It may be better to have the name of the facility in bold or even in blue bold in the white pages, and then take advantage of their 10 word special in the yellow pages that allows the facility's name to be listed in the yellow pages with 10 free words. This costs less than $30 per month and is much more cost-effective.

HOURS OF OPERATION

In order to be competitive in today's market place, hours of operation have to include morning hours and evening hours to accommodate the working client. Because most patients go to therapy three times per week, having at least three mornings and three evenings in the hours of operation is essential. An example of such a set-up may include 7 AM–11 AM and 4 PM–8 PM on Mondays (a split shift), 12 Noon–8 PM on Tuesdays and Thursdays, and 7 AM–3 PM on Wednesdays and Fridays. This is a 40-hour patient treatment week that accommodates both evening and daytime appointments. An owner of a business not only will work all those treatment hours, but will also spend at least 10–20 hours beyond that per week in marketing, promotion, and business activities for the business. As time goes on and more employees are brought into the business, the owner's time in treating patients may decrease and the time for business and marketing may increase. This is a plus and a minus in that individuals go to school to become clinicians, but as their career evolves they wind up spending less time in patient care and more time on business. The positive is that as more time is spent on promoting the business, it is hoped that business will continue to grow. It is essential that the business owner goes out, meets people in the business community, and meets physicians. Having other staff do this in addition is nice but it is essential that the owner spend the time to do these activities. In addition, as the business expands, a very dependable office manager can be hired to help with the paperwork, statistics, the number of patients seen per day or per week, the number of new evaluations, the number of cancellations and no-shows per clinician, payroll, and check writing. Because this is an important position in dealing with the financial aspects of the business, business owners tend to hire a family member whom they can depend upon to do these activities and who have some experience in this area.

MANAGED CARE

In today's health care industry, the future of the rehabilitation industry is questionable. Managed care involves, in most cases, an insurance company or its representatives "managing" the type, frequency, and duration of care received by its members in order to distribute total health care monies to providers in a more cost-efficient manner. Insurance companies are pushing to make more of a profit than they have in the past, and they are doing this by limiting the length of treatment for which they will reimburse, demanding outcome data, and decreasing the amount of reimbursement in order to demonstrate cost containment. This decreased reimbursement from insurance companies and higher operating costs, and increased taxes such as the energy tax, will significantly decrease the amount of profit that a business is able to produce in the future. Managed care is a reality. It is essential for the soon-to-be owner to not only advertise to case workers and insurance companies, but to also stay on top of potential contract negotiations and communicating with these insurers.

Information presented in this chapter was based upon business in the state of Delaware. Please contact your accountant/lawyer for specific modifications in your area.

Study Questions

1. Compare the various types of business structures. Identify what type of structure you would use and why.
2. If your business plan states that you will be the only clinician and that you will receive an average of two new patients per day (on a 5-day a week, 8-hour per day work schedule), and if the average patient came for 10 visits, how long would it take before you would be treating a maximized patient load? How many patients is a maximized load?
3. Continuing with your business plan from question #2 above, at the end of the first year what would be your total number of patient visits? If the average amount of money you were paid per visit is $52, what is your gross revenue for year 1? (Assume you are closed for a total of 10 business days for holidays and vacation.)
4. Using only the following large hypothetical expenses, give a list of your expenses and their hypothetical costs.

Expense	Hypothetical Cost
A. Rent	$25/sq. ft. (plan on a 1200–3200 sq. ft. facility, inclusive of all utilities except phone)
B. Employee Salary	One full-time clinician: $_____ One full-time manager: $_____
C. Employee Benefits	Assume 25% of the cost of employee salaries
D. Equipment	List and give approximate cost
E. Phone	Include yellow pages—minimum $100/month
F. Taxes and Licenses	List and give approximate costs
G. Advertising	First year could be 5%–10% of total cost, will decrease thereafter
H. Legal and Accounting Costs	Call for current rates
I. Supplies	List and give approximate costs
J. Loan Repayment	Call bank to find current interest rates
K. Other	List

5. Develop a business plan based on questions #2, #3, and #4 above. This plan should include predicted revenues, predicted expenses, amount of money you wish to loan, and how you plan on repaying the loan.

Suggested Readings

The Ernst & Young Guide to Financing for Growth. New York, NY: John Wiley & Sons Publishers; 1994

Withholding of Delaware Income Tax, Regulation, Employers Duties, and Withholding Tables. Division of Revenue, Dover, Delaware; 1995

Administrative Policy and Procedure

Jeff G. Konin, MEd, ATC, MPT

OBJECTIVES

Upon completion of this chapter, the student will be able to accomplish the following:

1. Define a policy and a procedure, and differentiate between the two

2. Become familiar with the goals and objectives of policies and procedures in clinical settings

3. Identify the different types of policies and procedures

4. Recognize different components that may comprise a policy and procedure manual in a clinical setting

Every organization that exists runs on a daily basis by some form of rules. These rules are what set the standards for consistent operational methods, and are commonly referred to as "policies and procedures." The type, extent, and enforcement of policies and procedures will vary from one facility to another.

By definition, a policy is "a definite course or method of action selected from among alternatives and in light of given conditions to guide and determine present and future decisions."[1] Although many clinical facilities have written policies regarding similar issues, the policies themselves should reflect the respected facility's goals and missions. For example, two neighboring clinical facilities may both have policies on tardiness to work. Facility A may take this as a serious concern and incorporate a strict policy against tardiness, whereas facility B may not think that tardiness to work is as much of a concern, and therefore they may have a lenient policy established.

The act or series of steps that is used to carry out a policy is referred to as the "procedure." Although a policy simply states what happens under an individual circumstance, it is the procedure that more clearly defines 1) who will carry out the process, 2) the time frame over which the action is implemented, and 3) the actual process of how the policy will be carried out.

In health care settings, an individual may find policy and procedure manuals that measure several inches in thickness. It behooves an employee to become familiar with the policies and procedures of his or her clinical facility.

GOALS AND OBJECTIVES OF THE POLICY AND PROCEDURE MANUAL

The main goal and objective of a policy and procedure manual is to provide for a decisive process that an individual may follow under various circumstances. This allows for consistency in the approach to decision-making processes and, more importantly, creates an environment in which equal opportunity exists.

When effective policies and procedures have been established in a clinical setting, the operation of the facility may run with less confusion and the employees may be able to better understand the daily decision-making process with respect to administrative affairs.

The goals and objectives of any policy and procedure manual should again reflect the beliefs of the organization with respect to administrative operations and client care. Because policies will affect the employer, the employees, and all those who receive service from the organization, they should be carefully thought out with an understanding of possible conflicts and repercussions.

Creation of a Policy and Procedure Manual

The process of devising a policy and procedure manual for a clinical setting can be a frustrating and tedious task. As mentioned earlier, many facilities maintain volumes of policies and procedures to ensure an algorithm-type pathway for each incident.

There are a number of steps that an individual must take when given the task of devising a policy and procedure manual. As expected, the initial process should include the formation of some kind of mission statement for the clinical facility. An example of a mission statement might be, "ATC Sports Medicine Clinic is devoted to providing the safest, most

---

Table 7-1

NATA Mission Statement

The mission of the National Athletic Trainers' Association is to enhance the quality of health care for the physically active and advance the profession of athletic training through education and research in the prevention, evaluation, management, and rehabilitation of injuries.

Reprinted with permission from *NATA Annual Report,* 1991-1992.

---

effective, and knowledgeable care to each and every client regardless of race, age, sex, or creed." This mission statement sets the tone for the development of the policies and procedures to follow. The mission statement that has been established by the NATA is outlined in Table 7-1.

It is also important to keep in mind any ethical and legal professional obligations that may need to be followed in order to practice and deliver a service to the public. For example, athletic trainers maintain professional standards of conduct as set forth by NATA. These standards should be included in the policy and procedure manual with appropriate referencing. In addition, several states legislate the practice of athletic training. These legislative documents should most certainly be included in the manual as well.

Because the organization and implementation of policies and procedures is complex and ultimately affects many individuals, input derived for the development of such a commodity should be taken from all of the people who may be influenced by the terms set forth. It is also a very good idea to receive input from legal counsel regarding the appropriateness of the terminology as well as the actual implementation of the policies and procedures themselves.

As will be discussed in Chapter 12, communication is an essential part of providing effective care. Having clearly written policies and procedures enhances the opportunity for positive communication among individuals when scenarios arise that must be resolved. By contrast, poorly written policies, or no policies at all, may lead to not only a breakdown in communication, but potential conflict among parties. In many instances, it is not until a conflict arises that an actual policy is then established as a result.

When establishing policies and procedures, an individual should always think permanence. Policies are not primarily intended to help an individual through a time of crisis, but instead are designed to establish order and rules for running the business.

Reliable policies and procedures can be beneficial in many ways. However, it is important to remember that establishing too many rules can actually be dissatisfying and provide for a very restrictive atmosphere in which to practice. Remember that different clinical facilities develop policies and procedures based on their individually respected missions and goals. Using the example of an employee being tardy to work, it is understandable how an overly aggressive policy can be unwarranted. It was mentioned that Facility A takes a very serious stand against employees who are late for work, and its policy states the following:

> No employee shall be tardy for work beyond 15 minutes. It will be procedure for the manager to assess each employee's time card at the end of the pay period. If it is found by a manager that an employee has punched in beyond 15 minutes of the expected time to begin work, then an automatic 5% will be deducted from the employee's next paycheck.

This is a very harsh example; however, it may be the only policy and procedure listed in Facility A's manual that addresses tardiness. If the reason for an employee being late was a very valid and understanding one, then a conflict would arise. The reason would either be completely ignored because the manager went strictly by the time card, or the manager would have to go against the policy to take the employee's stance on the issue.

A simple solution to the above procedure would be to add a plan that would give the employee an opportunity to express his or her situation either in writing or through a conference within a given time period. This would allow for the manager to make an educated and fair decision regarding the reason for tardiness as opposed to taking immediate harsh action. If, after reviewing the circumstances, the manager feels as though the reason for being tardy is not justified, then a pay deduction can still be implemented.

An additional stand on tardiness could also be added to the above policy and procedure stating that regardless of the reason, being tardy on more than two instances is subject to an automatic paycheck deduction. Now, understanding that unusual circumstances may arise, no employee is otherwise encouraged to show up for work late.

Because no clinical facility remains dormant with respect to its daily operations, it is important to continue to update policies on a regular basis. Doing so would allow for necessary changes that may have evolved as a result of demographics, legislation, employee concerns, and many other possible issues. Again, it is important to incorporate those affected by the changes in the review process.

To ensure effective communication of policies and procedures, it is recommended that employers have employees sign a form acknowledging that they have read, understood, and agreed to follow the terms of the policy and procedure manual. If possible, the employee should retain not only a copy of the signed form, but also of the manual itself.

Types of Policies and Procedures

In general, there are three types of policies and procedures: 1) administrative, 2) interdepartmental, and 3) departmental.[2] Each type is planned and documented specifically for the group of people that it is designed to serve.

Administrative policies and procedures are designed with the ultimate thought of preparing standards that will apply to a larger group of people who are typically employed in the same facility or work under the same management. These are the types of policies that one would often refer to when addressing concerns in the area of dress code, vacation requests, and maternity leave. They may also be established to define the procedures for daily operations such as patient billing, requests for medical records, and documentation.

Administrative policies and procedures may often be established as a result of requirements set forth by accreditation or regulation laws. When designing these policies and procedures to meet certain guidelines, consultations with experienced personnel who have successfully put together such work may be beneficial.

Interdepartmental policies are different than administrative policies in that they may not affect all parties working in the same facility or employed by the same company. These policies serve to organize the actions of different disciplines who may be working for the same common goal.

For example, an athletic trainer may treat a 67-year-old man who has recently undergone a total joint arthroplasty for his left shoulder. His insurance provider may require that he receive services from occupational therapy, physical therapy, and social services on a daily basis to meet the requirements for reimbursement during his hospital stay. It is therefore a responsibility of the said departments to communicate and coordinate their services to enable the patient to receive full benefits.

Many interdepartmental policies are written to include a multitude of disciplines. In a clinical setting where the philosophy is to always be friendly to all patients, its interdepartmental policy may be written to include departments such as physical therapy, secretarial, public relations, collections, and maintenance or janitorial.

Departmental policies and procedures are written specifically to address a group of people who may be performing different tasks than other groups within an organization. These people would still abide by all administrative and interdepartmental policies that affect their environment, but would also be held accountable for their own departmental guidelines.

Departmental policies and procedures are typically the most individualized as compared to interdepartmental and administrative. They are written to address the issues and concerns of a single department that may be unique and different to other departments.

An example of a departmental policy and procedure may be the cleaning and maintenance of whirlpools in a physical therapy department that is located in a large hospital. Because no other departments in the hospital perform whirlpool treatments, they would not be concerned with this policy. However, if this policy and the procedures for cleaning and maintaining a whirlpool are not correctly followed, the damage that may be done to the whirlpool and the potential risk of contaminating clients may directly affect all of those involved in the department in a variety of ways.

Contents of a Policy and Procedure Manual

It should be evident by now that there is a potential to write a policy for many, many issues. Even more so, for each policy that is written, numerous amounts of procedures could be applied to follow. Therefore, the contents of any policy and procedure manual should first and foremost be written specifically to address the needs of the individual facility at hand. By contrast, no policy and procedure manual should be designed with the goal of preparing to address every potential situation that may arise.[3]

Although no single manual that exists at any facility may be all-inclusive, Table 7-2 gives an example of an outline of a policy and procedure manual that may typically exist in a physical therapy clinic.

SUMMARY

Policies and procedures are used in clinical settings as a means to provide for consistency in the delivery of care as well as with daily administrative operations. The process of devising a policy and procedure manual is a complex task that should include the efforts of many individuals and be based on the goals and missions of the individual facility at hand.

The three types of policies and procedures are administrative, interdepartmental, and departmental. Policies and procedures should be complete with respect to these compo-

Table 7-2

Example Outline of a Policy and Procedure Manual for an Outpatient Physical Therapy Clinic

I. General Information
  A. Goals and Objectives
  B. Mission Statement
  C. Governing Laws
  D. Patient's Bill of Rights

II. Administrative Policies
  A. Orientation
  B. Organizational Structure
  C. Maintenance of Records
  D. Plan of Care
  E. Patient Billing
  F. Staff Attendance
  G. Release of Medical Records
  H. Quarterly and Yearly Reviews
  I. Hiring Practices
  J. Vacation Policy
  K. Benefits
  L. Payday Policy
  M. Incident Report
  N. Termination Policy
  O. Safety Considerations
    1. Access to Building
    2. OSHA Guidelines
  P. Inclement Weather
  Q. Hours of Operation
  R. Employee Parking
  S. Emergency Procedures
    1. Code
    2. Fire
  T. Sexual Harassment
  U. Use of Cafeteria

III. Interdepartmental Policies
  A. Staff Meetings
  B. Transfer of Patients
  C. Patient Scheduling
  D. Maintenance of Records
  E. Patient Referral
  F. Documentation

IV. Departmental Policies
  A. Job Descriptions
  B. Scheduling of Patients
  C. Maintenance of Records
  D. Employee Evaluations
  E. Licensure
  F. Dress Code
  G. Incident Report
  H. Safety Considerations
    1. Soiled Linen
    2. Infection Control
    3. Equipment Repair
    4. OSHA Guidelines
  I. Equipment
    1. Whirlpool
    2. Ultrasound
    3. Paraffin
    4. Electrical Modalities
  J. Documentation
  K. Purchasing
  L. Delivery of Packages

nents. Even though the contents of a policy and procedure manual may not be all-inclusive, it should at the very least address the common issues and concerns of the daily operations of a department.

Study Questions

1. Define a policy and a procedure, and explain their relationship.
2. What are the goals and objectives of policies and procedures?
3. What steps should an individual take when given the task of devising a policy and procedure manual?

4. List the three types of policies and procedures and explain the differences among them. Give an example of each as it relates to a hospital setting.

5. Think of an issue that you would consider important enough to be included in a policy and procedure manual. If you were devising the manual, how would you write the policy, and what procedures would be set forth to enforce your policy?

References

1. *Webster's New Collegiate Dictionary.* Springfield, Mass: Merriam Webster Inc.; 1994.

2. Nosse LJ, Friberg DG. *Management Principles for Physical Therapists.* Baltimore, Md: Williams & Wilkins; 1992.

3. *American Institute of Small Business.* Minneapolis, Minn: AISB Publishing;1990;1.

Suggested Readings

Anderson GR, Anderson GVA. *Health Care Ethics.* Rockville, Md: Aspen; 1987.

Commission on the Accreditation of Rehabilitation Facilities. Standards manual for organizations serving people with disabilities. Tucson, Ariz: Commission of Accreditation of Rehabilitation Facilities; 1990.

Mathews J. *Practice Issues in Physical Therapy.* Thorofare, NJ: SLACK Inc; 1989.

National Athletic Trainers' Association Annual Report, Dallas, Tex, 1991–1992.

Payton OD, Pzer MN, Nelson CE. *Patient participation in program planning: a manual for therapists.* Philadelphia, Pa: FA Davis Publishers; 1990.

The Dartnell Personnel Administration Handbook, 3rd ed. Chicago, Ill: Dartnell Press; 1985.

Fiscal Management

Ronnie P. Barnes, MS, ATC

OBJECTIVES

Upon completion of this chapter, the student will be able to accomplish the following:

1. Understand the importance of fiscal management in clinical athletic training settings

2. Recognize the objectives of business as it relates to clinical athletic training

3. Discuss financial planning in terms of athletic health care

4. Differentiate between various types of budgets used in clinical settings

5. Recognize inventory as a vital component in preparing a budget

Health care professionals often neglect to improve their knowledge base in business. Most caregivers enter the health care field because they enjoy helping the sick and injured. The concept of money and helping is somewhat foreign to them. Many health care professionals are extremely poor at conducting business. Physicians are often referred to by accountants and money managers as the worst business people. It is important to understand basic accounting principals and overall fiscal management if one intends to be successful in today's health care market.

THE BUSINESS OF SPORTS MEDICINE

As health care professionals move from entry level positions to the positions of experienced practitioners, the level of responsibility changes. Recognizing that sports medicine operates in a business environment is sometimes a harsh reality. Financial analysis becomes part of the job description for those individuals in leadership roles within the business. It is important for any professional to understand the objectives of business to really understand business. Six components universally express the objectives of all business operations. The health care professional may not be responsible for each objective, but is affected by them all.

1. **Sales**—In private practice, sales represent revenue from patient visits. In the sports setting, sales are determined by fan attendance at sporting events, revenue from licensed apparel, and concessions.
2. **Costs**—In all sports medicine settings, costs represent operating expenses. This includes all overhead, salaries, facility management, travel, and other organizational expenses. The costs are expressed in business as variable and fixed.
3. **Profits**—Profits reflect the organization's ability to use its assets to make money. Profits can be further described as the amount of revenue remaining after all of the expenses of the organization have been paid.
4. **Revenue**—Revenue is the total of all of the monetary receipts of an enterprise. Sales of service, merchandise, and product produced revenue. Revenue can also be stated as income from earnings from interest, dividends, rents, and wages.
5. **Return on Investment**—This represents the ratio between the capital outlay, or monies invested to run the organization, and the revenue collected on that capital outlay. Negative returns on investments represent losses. Positive returns on investment represent profits. This is usually expressed in percents.
6. **Growth Earnings**—This shows growth in revenue (earnings) above expenses over time. Companies like to see an increase in revenue from one year to the next. It does not necessarily indicate that the company is making a profit, but it does indicate an increase or decrease in the movement of goods and services.

Meeting these objectives is the goal of every organization. Understanding these objectives will assist the athletic trainer in working with his or her organization in financial planning and budgeting.

ACCOUNTING

Accounting involves collecting financial information that is important to the survival of a business organization. University athletic departments, high school sports programs, and private sports medicine clinics are all businesses. The businesses spend and collect money, or revenue, in the operational processes. Accounting is the scorecard that defines what financial resources are available and helps determine how monies should be spent. In the private sector, finances are a major focus to the employer because the business operates to make a profit. Even nonprofit organizations operate to make profits and not to lose money. Those profits allow them to conduct programs.

Economics play a material role in sports programs at all levels. High schools that play in state championships and college teams that earn berths to football bowl games and basketball finals fare better financially than their counterparts that finish in the league cellar. Profits gained from this success help to fund the least revenue-sponsored sports and the institution's sports medicine program. Accounting determines how much money will be available for the provision of health care.

Accountants and business managers are concerned with precise, reliable, and timely financial information. Health practitioners gather financial information relevant to the department. This information helps to construct the budget and determines how the revenue allotted to the medical department will be spent. Learning how to present this data to the bean counters in a useful manner is essential to management. Understanding financial terms and jargon will aid in speaking the language that accountants comprehend.

The present health care market place is burdened by inflation and spiraling increases in health care costs. Efficient financial health care management is crucial in the continuation of quality health care. This requires scientific accounting and fiscal controls. As a result, there have been numerous developments in the use and procedures of accounting in health care. Capitation in health care reimbursement and managed care systems are both evolutions designed to better control and account for expenditures in health care. In simple terms, the health care dollar is being stretched as far as it can stretch, and accounting tracks these dollars every cent of the way.

Computerized accounting is very helpful in financial management. Contemporary software packages allow one to collect, review, and utilize this information in innovative and useful ways. Department supervisors are able to review computerized financial summaries on a regular basis. These documents outline the financial information relevant to providing health care, and allow the professional to react to financial changes much sooner than in previous decades.

FINANCIAL PLANNING

Financial planning is a continuous look into the fiscal future of an organization. Fiscal management requires constant and continuous planning. Planning galvanizes a health care professional's knowledge of health care delivery and the costs of providing that care. Just as an athletic trainer would formulate goals and objectives for a sick or injured athlete, he or she must consider the goals and objectives of a company, institution, or team. The health of a business organization is dependent upon thorough planning. Sports medicine departments must constantly juggle the cost of services and quality care. Proper planning for event coverage, supplies, and manpower can preserve quality of care by optimizing the available resources. Providing health care for athletes at a college or high school can be expensive. Because the organization is usually not reimbursed by an insurance company or some other third party, planning is important to predict the cost of providing care to each participant on each team. Expendable supplies such as tape, bandages, and sports beverages represent an expense that must be included in a plan to avoid depletion. Successful planning permits the medical professional to render care on a quality basis from one athlete to another throughout the year.

Budgets in Sports Medicine

Budgets are instruments that illustrate expenses and revenue in a particular department. Preparing a budget requires a coordination of resources and expenditures. It also requires a global understanding of all expenses related to providing health care in the sports medicine setting. All overhead, including salaries and other employee expenses, are stated in the budget. Every expense that is authorized by the sports medicine department is debited from its budget. Budgets should be designed to predict the needs of the department and eliminate excess waste. The first time budget preparer will benefit from reviewing historical department expenditures from previous years.

Budgets are planned in coordination with the sports medicine department head, the athletic director or chairperson, and the business manager. Most budgets are reviewed on an annual basis; however, some budgets are projected for periods of up to 3 years with increases built in for inflation along the way. Extended budgets should be monitored on a quarterly basis to predict hidden or unexpected expenses. Adjustments can be made along the way to compensate for these surprises.

Budget projections provide a financial picture for the sports medicine department. They will show expected revenue and expenses, assets, and liabilities. Careful and precise planning in developing a budget allows for a smooth and functional operation of the sports medicine department. Deficits in operational expenses are usually related to poor planning or unrealistically low allocations of revenue.

Types of Budgets

In his textbook, *Management Strategies in Athletic Training*, Richard Ray describes nine different types of budgets:
1. Spending ceiling model or incremental model
2. Spending reductions
3. Zero-based budgeting
4. Planning, budgeting, and evaluation
5. Fixed budgeting
6. Variable budgeting
7. Lump sum budgeting
8. Line item budgeting
9. Performance budgeting

Each budget type requires extensive planning and working with management in developing flexibility in expenditures. Depending upon the financial solvency of the organization and its accounting sophistication, any of these budgets may be utilized.

Line Item Budgeting

A line item budget allocates revenue in broad categories related to the operation of the sports medicine department (Table 8-1). Lump sums are allocated for each category. Flexibility to move allocated money from one category to the next is optimal but not always permitted. For instance, if travel has been over-allocated and there is a shortage of revenue in supplies, it would be beneficial to have the flexibility to move revenue to the depleted line item. This flexibility usually can be negotiated with the business manager if the business is solvent.

Line item budgets require the maximum amount of planning, but they are among the easiest to understand and operate. The line item preparation begins with a review of the previous year's spending in each category. Justification for increases should be well documented. Broad categories such as travel are preferred over more specific categories like airplane, train, taxi, and personal car. Broad categories allow for expenditures regardless of the form of travel. Salaries, expendable supplies, and the overall costs of medical services are all categorized. Quality medical care must always be given prime consideration regardless of the budget type.

The budget can be viewed as an evolving document that may require the addition or deletion of line items from year to year. The following items can be examined at a budget meeting scheduled annually with the administration:

1. Discuss unexpected expenses or line item shifts from the previous year.
2. Study and predict trends that may precipitate increases in operational expenses.
3. Build in additional revenue for price escalations for goods that may cost more due to inflation.
4. Look for areas in the budget that may have been unrealistically shorted or underfunded and areas of excess that may be shifted to another category.
5. Ask for monthly or quarterly reports that will help in planning operational changes.
6. Insist on line items for books, periodicals, and continuing education. The athletic training profession mandates continuing education credits. Include revenue for travel, lodging, and expenses for all members of the department for continuing education.

Inventory Control

All businesses have expenses related to expendable items, consumable items, or items in stock for retail purposes. These items are purchases and they are stored until utilized and sold. Inventory is a common element in retail, wholesale, manufacturing, and service. For example, sports medicine is a service. Athletic tape, bandages, alcohol, and scissors are purchased in clinics and stored as inventory until utilized in providing health care. Budgets and historical use patterns determine the quantity of each item stored in inventory.

Inventory control is the counting, recording, and safe storage of items purchased. A sound accounting of the inventory on a monthly or quarterly basis ensures that the inventory will always contain optimal levels of supplies in economical quantities. It also ensures proper turnover of inventory and reduces excessive shrinkage. There are sometimes unexpected demands on inventory or shipping delays that can be avoided by proper inventory accounting. Major software vendors sell spreadsheet and database programs that can be tailored to meet the needs of an inventory control system.

Inventory should be stored in a safe, securable space. Climate control may be necessary for some products to avoid spoilage. Pilferage can reduce inventory and adversely affect the budget. Items in the inventory, such as crutches and elastic bandages, can be reused by the athletic patient population. A check-out system to track these and other reusable items is cost-efficient. Avoid maintaining excess inventory that must be discarded because

Table 8-1
Sample Line Item Budget
NEW YORK FOOTBALL GIANTS, INC.
FINANCIAL STATEMENTS FOR FISCAL YEAR

February 28, 1995 — November 1994

Description	November					Year to Date				
	1994 Actual	1994 Budget	1993 Actual	Variance to Budget	Variance to 1993	1994	Budget	1993	Budget Variance	1993 Variance
Medical and Trainers:										
Basic Compensation	17,199	17,821	17,008	(622)	191	160,728	160,388	157,948	340	2,780
Bonuses—Year-End						0	0	0	0	0
Bonuses—Playoff						0	0	0	0	0
Contribution to Pre-59er Plan						0	0	0	0	0
Payroll Taxes						0	0	0	0	0
Workers Compensation						0	0	0	0	0
Medical Insurance						0	0	0	0	0
Air Transportation	2,624	500	1,104	2,124	1,520	15,739	8,200	7,450	7,539	8,289
Ground Transportation—Auto	93	0	164	93	(71)	1,543	3,050	401	(1,507)	1,142
Staff Clothing Purchases		0		0	0	0	400	174	(400)	(174)
Equipment Rentals		0	32	0	(32)	2,338	1,900	3,175	438	(837)
Meals & Entertainment		0		0	0	2,018	250	1,807	1,768	211
Hotel Room Charges		0		0	0	3,246	1,750	1,412	1,496	1,834
Travel Costs —Other		0	64	0	(64)	254	200	79	54	175
Physicians	3,147	23,000	9,666	(23,000)	(6,519)	214,599	245,600	229,379	(31,001)	(14,780)
Hospitals	(1,456)	23,000	2,774	(23,000)	(4,230)	74,658	87,000	82,070	(12,342)	(7,412)

continued

Table 8-1 (continued)

Sample Line Item Budget
NEW YORK FOOTBALL GIANTS, INC.
FINANCIAL STATEMENTS FOR FISCAL YEAR

February 28, 1995   November 1994

Description	1994 Actual	1994 Budget	1993 Actual	November Variance to Budget	November Variance to 1993	1994	Budget	1993	Year to Date Budget Variance	Year to Date 1993 Variance
Drugs & Supplies	1,050	4,800	10,924	(4,800)	(9,874)	91,948	81,200	79,565	10,748	12,383
Dental		0	173	0	0	0	250	475	(250)	(475)
Eye Care	(60)	100		(100)	(233)	2,845	4,650	4,441	(1,805)	(1,596)
Braces	864	100	1,162	(100)	(298)	10,246	5,300	7,033	4,946	3,213
Disability Premiums		0		0	0	0	0	0	0	0
Other		0	8	0	(8)	3,304	1,950	1,359	1,354	1,954
Telephone		50		50	0	0	400	0	(400)	0
Delivery Costs	5,202	500	1,038	(500)	4,164	14,141	7,050	7,169	7,091	6,972
Per Diem Allowances	54	0		0	54	1,078	400	578	678	500
Subscriptions	490	0	524	0	(34)	980	600	1,273	380	(293)
Living & Family Moving					0	9,470	0	0	9,470	9,470
Departmental Supplies	95				95	1,071	0	0	1,071	1,071
Repairs & Maintenance				0	0	455	0	0	455	455
Miscellaneous Expenses	580	400	1,249	(400)	(669)	15,381	5,000	7,477	10,381	7,904
TOTAL Medical and Trainers	29,882	70,271	45,890	(50,355)	(16,008)	626,042	615,538	593,265	10,504	32,777

it is outdated or obsolete. These practices waste money that may be better spent rendering health care. A sound system of inventory purchase, storage, and inventory control reduces costs to the organization. Proper planning helps the clinical manager decide the appropriate amount of supplies to be ordered for the buying period. Inventory carries the hidden expenses of shipping, storage, insurance, and taxes. This inventory must be viewed as cash on the shelf. Unnecessary purchasing and unscrupulous utilization erodes the budget and affects the efficiency of the health care program. Ideally, an inventory accounting program should be developed to order new products only when certain levels are reached in the inventory of each item. This ensures fresh products and allows the business to invest its money in a bank and not on the inventory shelf.

Bids and Requests for Quotation

Several suppliers should be contacted to compare prices and delivery forms when an order is placed. Maintaining a library of catalogs with descriptions and catalog numbers for specifications is helpful in the bid procedure. Price alone is not the sole reason for ordering from a vendor. Service and delivery, as well as providing the exact products specified, is very important. When the clinical manager seeks bids, he or she should send each vendor a request for quotation clearly outlining product specifications, including brands and catalog numbers. All requests for quotes from vendors should be identical and be computed on a common basis (e.g., units, dozens, lots). Information regarding costs of packaging and shipping should be requested also. Quotations may be solicited by telephone or they may be distributed on standard forms through the mail. It is important for the manager to be very specific about specifications and quantities on the quotation forms.

Clinical managers should be aware of new suppliers and products that can meet the clinic's needs at lower costs. Sports medicine vendors are competitive and will quote their best prices when they know the purchaser maintains the option to buy elsewhere. Always have a back-up supplier to protect against a sole provider raising prices or not stocking the items needed for a program. Large quantities should be purchased when discounts are available. Vendors often give price breaks as the quantity of an item ordered increases. The clinical manager should constantly try to improve the terms and conditions of the clinic's purchases. Revenue saved on supplies can be utilized in other areas of the budget.

Receiving Shipments

In most instances, the supplies ordered will be shipped to the institution or facility. Because much can happen to a shipment between the time it leaves the shipper's loading dock and the time it arrives at the facility, the clinical manager should know how to minimize freight problems.

At the time of delivery, the count should be verified to make certain that the amount shipped has been delivered. This number may vary from the amount ordered because often items are back ordered, or sent later, when the vendor does not have the product in stock. The Bill of Lading is a document given to the receiver of goods by the tracking company at the time of delivery. This document should be reviewed carefully and checked to verify that all of the numbers match. If there is a discrepancy or the product is damaged, the clinical manager should call the vendor immediately while the trucker is in his or her presence. If the vendor is not available, delivery may be refused, or copious notes should be made on the Bill of Lading to indicate the shipping problem. One copy should be given to the trucker, and a copy for the clinic's records should be kept. The driver should sign both copies.

All cartons should be opened and inspected for damage to contents immediately after delivery. Retain any damaged items and call the vendor or carrier to report the damage and request an inspection. Vendors will generally accept return of the items at their expense and settle the damage problems directly with the carrier. Items should never be returned to the vendor without written or verbal permission to do so. Items can be misplaced at shipping facilities and this can create more problems and expenses.

SUMMARY

Since the practice of providing sound, competent health care has developed into an operational business from all aspects of practice, it is incumbent upon the clinical athletic trainer to become more familiar with the process. Understanding the objectives of a business and how they relate to the preparation of developing a budget on a regular basis are skills that every athletic trainer should possess regardless of his or her level of clinical practice. It is the potential success of fiscal management that ensures one's employment in a particular facility. The clinical athletic trainer who recognizes early on in his or her career that the delivery of health care is a business that can be run by any and all providers is sure to place him- or herself one step ahead of the rest of the field.

Study Questions

1. Explain why sound fiscal management is essential to a clinical facility.
2. Differentiate between sales, costs, profits, revenue, return on investment, and growth earnings as they relate to business.
3. As a clinical athletic trainer in charge of inventory, you realize that certain popular items appear to be disappearing from your stock without proper documentation. What measures should you take to assess the whereabouts of these items? How could you ensure a better system to protect these products?
4. As the newly appointed director of a clinical setting, you have been given the task of developing the budget for the upcoming year. First, what steps would you take to begin your planning? Second, how would you determine which items or expenditures are necessary versus those that could be eliminated?
5. In follow-up to question 4, prepare an actual line item budget for the upcoming fiscal year. Be sure to include revenues as well as expenses, and attempt to demonstrate how your facility would create a positive return on its investment.

Suggested Readings

Eisen P. *Accounting 1994*. 3rd ed. Hauppauge, NY: Barron's Educational Series, Inc.

Finnely RG. *Basics of Budgeting*. New York, NY: American Management Association; 1994.

Ray R. *Management Strategies in Athletic Training*. Champaign, Ill: Human Kinetics Publishers; 1994.

Shiry JK, Siegel JG. *Budgeting Basics & Beyond*. Englewood Cliffs, NJ: Prentice Hall; 1994.

Williamson AD, ed. *Business Terms 1993*. Boston, Mass: Harvard Business School Press.

Reimbursement for Health Care Services

Mark S. De Carlo, MHA, PT, SCS, ATC

OBJECTIVES

Upon completion of this chapter, the student will be able to accomplish the following:

1. Be familiar with the history of health care reimbursement

2. Understand the rationale for changes in the American health care system and how this has affected reimbursement

3. Recognize common insurance terminology, including different types of insurance plans, corresponding terminology and diagnostic and procedural coding

4. Know the specific steps involved with submitting an insurance claim in order to secure reimbursement for services

5. Have some understanding of the involvement of the National Athletic Trainers' Association in securing reimbursement from third party payers

In the early 1960s, social philosophy in America emphasized that all citizens were entitled to the best possible health care services with equal access for everyone. This philosophy of entitlement was quite evident in public policy of that particular time in history. Landmark health care legislation was passed by the federal government, which was primarily intended to meet the health care needs of poor, elderly, and disabled citizens.[1,2]

Title XVIII of the Social Security Act was enacted in 1965, creating the Medicare System. Primary legislative support for the passage of Medicare came from organized labor, not from the health care system. This emphasized the significant political clout of labor unions and the fact that at that time the American economy was industrial based. An administrative provision of the Medicare legislation, which ultimately had a tremendous economic impact on our health care system as a whole, allowed for provider reimbursement based on costs. This was in contrast to established fee schedules that were in place at the time.[2,3]

Around this time, Title XIX of the Social Security Act created the Medicaid system. This was established as a state administered program to provide health care services to poor, elderly, and disabled citizens not covered under any other health care plan, including Medicare. Medicaid mandated a core number of services, with the individual states maintaining the option of providing additional services as appropriate. Expenses associated with providing Medicaid services are shared between federal and state government. The establishment of government-sponsored health care payment systems positioned federal and state government as a driving force behind the growth of the American health care industry and the ongoing increase in health care costs over the years.[2,3]

Reimbursement for health care services has traditionally been provided through four primary sources including: 1) federal government, 2) state and local government, 3) business by providing health insurance to employees, and 4) personal household income and philanthropy. Following the introduction of Medicare and Medicaid in 1965, the expenditures for health care services allocated to each group has continually changed. Business and government have been responsible for an increasingly higher percentage of health care costs than any of the other groups.[4]

Blue Cross/Blue Shield implemented a reimbursement system in the 1960s that paid providers for services based on usual, customary, and reasonable rates. This replaced the use of standardized fee schedules that had been used for many years prior to the new system. Reimbursement for Medicare services when the program was first implemented was on a cost-plus basis. This system involved paying the provider for the cost of services and an additional amount to cover such expenditures as depreciation of capital equipment. Payment under the traditional Blue Cross/Blue Shield indemnity system and Medicare were not tied to a specific fee schedule and there were no specific built-in constraints on utilization of services. This type of payment system promotes providers and recipients of health care to use the philosophy that "if a little is good, more is better."[1,4]

A CHANGING HEALTH CARE SYSTEM

The American health care system has undergone tremendous change since the implementation of Medicare and Medicaid in 1965. It became apparent soon after the implementation of these programs that the costs associated with providing such services would eventually be a financial burden on the federal budget. In addition, with the introduction of usual and customary reimbursement for traditional indemnity insurance such as Blue Cross and Blue Shield, businesses who paid for health care for their employees would eventually be financially drained by the system.[1]

Many of the changes that have occurred in our health care system are directly related to the ongoing effort to control spiraling costs. A number of significant changes within the system resulted from the various financial constraints inherent to the overall system. The single greatest impetus for change was the rapid and uncontrolled increase in health care costs. The push for change came from a number of sources outside the health care industry, including the federal government and business community. Health care providers at the time, including physicians and hospitals, were quite content with the system. Services could be provided to needy patients without restrictions on reimbursement.

One of the more significant changes included a philosophical shift in the delivery of health care services. The traditional view by most citizens was that health care was a basic human right. Through the 1970s with the increasing federal tax burden and budget deficit, the American people began to struggle with the premise of equal access to the best quality health care services for all citizens. The foundation for this change in social philosophy centered on the continually increasing tax burden from such a system as it was structured at the time.

The economic burden of providing health care services was on the federal government and the business community. Their initial efforts were driven by the need to control health care costs with the underlying philosophy that "increased consumer choice, more efficient health care providers, and lower costs" were the answer to many of the problems facing the system. Cost-containment efforts were meant to significantly shift the power base of the health care delivery system and provide a major restructuring of provider reimbursement. The primary methods of modifying the system at that time included shifting the risk for health care expenditures from the payer (federal government and businesses) to the providers and beneficiaries of care. This was accomplished through a gradual implementation of increased premiums, deductibles, and copayments as well as the introduction of managed care plans.[5-8]

Changes in the early 1980s prompted revolutionary modifications in our health care system. During this time period, America continued the evolutionary reformation from an industrial to a service-based economy. As a result of this change, labor unions had significantly less political control and had less influence on the extent of health care benefits for their members. Providers were forced to shift cost to government and corporate payers in order to ease the burden of providing care to the underinsured and uninsured. As a result, businesses faced tremendous increases in health care premiums. Health care expenditures made it difficult for federal and state government to meet all of its obligations including other entitlement programs such as welfare.[5]

One of the most significant changes to the Medicare system since its inception occurred in 1983. The Social Security Act of 1983 dramatically altered reimbursement for inpatient health care services. This legislative change eliminated cost-plus reimbursement and replaced it with a prospective payment system. With this form of reimbursement, all Medicare patients that are admitted to the hospital as an inpatient are assigned to a diagnostic related group (DRG). This assignment is made based on the primary diagnosis, with each DRG having a set description of the clinical condition and an established preset care plan to meet its medical needs. Reimbursement for each DRG is set in advance with the provider getting paid this preset fee, regardless of what it actually costs to provide the care. A profit is realized if the costs associated with providing services stay below the preset rate. However, if the cost of care exceeds the preset rate, the provider loses money. The principle focus of the prospective payment system was to begin sharing the risk associated with the provision of health care, with both the payer and the provider assuming some degree of risk.[1]

It was initially believed that the prospective payment system would, as a cost cutting measure, result in a decrease in the utilization of ancillary health care services such as physical and occupational therapy. However, the relationship between timely hospital discharge and appropriate rehabilitation immediately became recognized. An increased demand for rehabilitative services in skilled nursing facilities and home care settings also occurred. Hospital diversification and vertical integration of entire health care systems significantly increased inpatient, outpatient, and long-term care programs. As other ancillary health service providers, such as athletic trainers, attempt to secure third party reimbursement for professional services, it is imperative that they realize the importance of establishing a presence in the health care system. This includes establishing a set educational curriculum and certification or licensing process, demonstrating clinical competence, and documenting clinical outcomes.[9]

As the federal government sought to limit health care expenditures in the 1980s through the implementation of the prospective payment system, businesses attempted to control their financial risk through support of the managed care model. Managed care organizations bridge the gap between providers and consumers, serving to ultimately control utilization and cost of health care services.[1,10-12]

The health maintenance organization (HMO) model establishes a set premium based on an estimate of what it will cost to provide services to the beneficiaries of the plan. Businesses are able to save money through this kind of arrangement through less premium dollars. The HMO attempts to control utilization of services and costs in a number of different ways. The principle construct of the managed care model is to control access to care through the use of a gatekeeper. A primary care physician serves as gatekeeper. The plan participants must seek authorization from the gatekeeper for any specialty services beyond that of primary care. The HMO model will often provide certain diagnostic services, medications, and durable medical equipment and supplies directly or contract for such services at a discounted rate. In addition, the managed care program will often include capitation or discounted arrangements with specialty providers and hospitals. With capitation, the provider is paid a set fee for each covered life each month. It then becomes the provider's responsibility to provide all of the necessary care regardless of the actual costs to provide that care. Capitation is another example of how risk in a managed care environment is shared between all participants.[1,12]

The changing health care system of the 1990s has continued to affect providers at all levels and has left no one immune to change. Utilization control has extended to providers of rehabilitation services by limiting patients' access to care, increasing documentation and clinical outcomes requirements, and ultimately increasing accountability to consumers and payers. In spite of the recognized role of the rehabilitation specialist, it is not expected that his or her position will remain as it has been in the past. The profession as a whole must be willing to make the necessary changes to effectively deal with health reform. Health care professionals have spent little time assimilating comparable patient databases, management systems, and standardized treatment protocols or documenting patient protocols. Health care reform is demanding that providers be more accountable for their professional performance and more cost effective in providing patient treatment. Health care providers will continue to see the demand from third party payers for documenting the need and efficacy of treatment while keeping the cost of care within payer defined limits.[1,13-15]

INSURANCE TERMINOLOGY

A principle factor relating to successful reimbursement for health care services involves a detailed understanding of insurance terminology. Having achieved a baseline of knowledge relating to insurance, it then becomes necessary to understand procedural coding of insurance claims as well as diagnostic coding that is essential for accurate relaying of diagnostic data between the provider and the third party payer for reimbursement.

Insurance Plans

Indemnity Plan

An indemnity plan is a commercial fee-for-service plan that permits its beneficiaries to seek care without restriction and reimburses providers on a fee-for-service basis. There are generally no incentives to control utilization or costs with this type of plan.[16,17]

Health Maintenance Organization (HMO)

An HMO is a prepaid health care provider group practice serving a specific geographic area. Based on federal regulations, in order to qualify as an HMO the organization must have: 1) an organized system for providing health care or ensuring health care delivery in a geographic area, 2) an agreed upon set of basic and supplemental health maintenance and treatment services, and 3) a voluntary enrolled group of people.[16,17]

Preferred Provider Organization (PPO)

A PPO is a group plan in which participating physician providers have signed contracts to provide exclusive care for plan members at specific contract fees. The reimbursement rate is discounted below that of regular fee-for-service arrangements.[16,17]

Medicare

Medicare is the largest medical benefits program in the country. It is federally funded and administered by the Health Care Finance Administration. Plan beneficiaries include all people age 65 and over receiving social security benefits and all people receiving social security disability benefits.[16,17]

Medicaid

Medicaid is a combined federal and state program designed to provide health care services to the poor and medically indigent citizens. People who qualify for Medicaid include those receiving Supplemental Security Income or Aid to Families with Dependent Children Benefits, as well as citizens whose income falls below the national poverty level.[16,17]

Corresponding Terminology

- **Allowable Charge:** The maximum amount, according to the individual policy, that insurance will pay for each procedure or service performed.
- **Beneficiary:** A person eligible to receive the benefits of a specific policy or program.
- **Benefits:** Services that an insurer, government agency, or health care plan offers to pay for an insured individual.
- **Capitation:** A method of payment for health care services in which the health care provider is paid a set fee per member in a fixed period of time, not based on types or number of services provided.
- **Case Management Services:** The process in which the attending physician or agent coordinates the care given to a patient by other health care providers and/or community organizations.
- **Claim:** A form sent to an insurance company requesting payment for covered medical expenses. Information includes the insured's name and address, procedure codes, diagnostic codes, charges, and date of service.
- **Clean Claim:** A filed claim with all of the necessary information that may be immediately processed.
- **Contract:** A legally binding agreement between an insurance company and a physician describing the duties of both parties.
- **Copayment:** A provision in an insurance policy requiring the policy holder to pay a specified percentage of each medical claim.
- **Customary Fees:** The average fee charged for a specified service or procedure in a defined geographic area.
- **Deductible:** The amount owed by the insured on a yearly basis before the insurance company will begin to pay for services rendered.
- **Dependent:** A person legally eligible for benefits based on his or her relationship with the policy holder.
- **Exclusions:** Specified medical services, disorders, treatments, diseases, and durable medical equipment that is listed as uncovered or not reimbursable in an insurance policy.
- **Explanation of Benefits (EOB):** An insurance report accompanying all claim payments that explains how the insurance company processed a claim.
- **Fee Schedule:** A comprehensive listing of the maximum payment amount that an insurance company will allow for specified medical procedures performed on a beneficiary of the plan.
- **Gatekeeper:** The primary care physician assigned by the insurer that oversees the medical care rendered to a patient and initiates all specialty and ancillary services.
- **Managed Care:** A system in which costs are controlled by closely monitoring health care provider's treatment, requiring preauthorization for hospital admissions, surgeries, and referrals to specialists.
- **Participating Provider:** A health care provider who has entered into a contract with an insurance company to provide medical services to the beneficiaries of a plan. The provider agrees to accept the insurance company's approved fee and will only bill the patient for the deductible, copayment, and uncovered services.
- **Policy Holder:** The person who takes out the medical insurance policy.
- **Premium:** A periodic payment made to an insurance company by an individual pol-

icy holder or employer, in the case of group coverage, to pay for health care coverage.

- **Third Party Administrator:** An independent organization that collects premiums, pays claims, and provides administrative services within a health care plan.
- **UCR Allowable Charge:** Usual, customary, and reasonable charge that represents the maximum amount an insurance company will pay for a given service based on geographical averages.

Diagnostic Coding

Accurate medical insurance coding is an essential component of an insurance claim and is necessary in order to secure reimbursement for services. All diagnostic codes are obtained from the International Classification of Diseases (ICD). The Health Care Financing Administration (HCFA) and the private insurance industry require coding of all diagnoses. Submitted claims are generally checked via computer databases to ensure that payments are made only for the procedures that are medically necessary and related to the diagnosis.[16,17]

Procedural Coding

An additional factor that relates to the submission of a clean claim and successful reimbursement involves procedural coding. Current Procedural Terminology (CPT) is a nationally standardized system of coding that involves using five digit numbers to identify specific medical services. As with diagnostic coding, third party payers perform a computerized check of available data systems to ensure reimbursement is made from procedures that are accurately matched to a diagnosis that requires such services.[16,17]

SPECIFIC STEPS FOR SUBMITTING AN INSURANCE CLAIM

Successful reimbursement is dependent upon a number of factors, including a clear understanding of insurance terminology as well as diagnostic and procedural coding. With this information as a foundation, one must then comprehend the steps necessary in submitting a clean claim to the insurance company or managed care organization in order to obtain reimbursement for professional services provided.

An accurate and complete patient registration form (Figure 9-1) must be obtained from the patient as a first step in submitting an insurance claim for reimbursement. It is with this information that a medical record and patient account can be established. Many health care facilities have computerized medical records and accounting systems for such purposes. Various software programs are available that include a multitude of capabilities. It is possible to establish a medical billing system on personal computers for smaller offices and move up to a main frame system for larger offices.

The step-by-step process involved in submitting an insurance claim for reimbursement is as follows:

Step 1: Complete the Patient Encounter Form

The patient encounter form (Figure 9-2) is used by the health care provider in documenting the services provided to the patient at the time of his or her visit. In addition, the

Doctor _____

Org. Date _____   Print Date

Medical Rec. # _____   Fin. Class

==
    PATIENT INFORMATION
==

Name _____   SS# _____   Sex (M/F) __

Address _____   Home Phone _____   _____

City/St/Zip _____   Birth Date _____   Age ___

Employer _____   Address _____

City/St/Zip _____   Phone _____   _____

Nearest
Relative _____   Address _____

City/St/Zip _____   Phone _____   _____

School _____   Phone _____   _____

School Address _____

Coach _____   Trainer _____

Family Doctor _____   Phone _____

Address _____   City/St/Zip _____

==
    GUARANTOR INFORMATION
    (Complete this section if patient is a minor or student)
==

Guarantor Name _____   SS# _____

Address _____   Home Phone _____   _____

City/St/Zip _____   Work Phone _____   _____

Employer _____   Address _____
City/St/Zip _____

==
    INSURANCE INFORMATION
==

Insurance Co. _____   ID# _____

Address _____   Grp# _____

Insured's Name _____

==
    INJURY INFORMATION
==

Injury Area _____   Injury Date _____

Is it sports related? __ Yes __ No   Sport _____

Is it work related? __ Yes __ No

Who referred you? __ Coach __ Trainer __ AD __ Friend __ Yellow Pages __ Relative

Referring Dr. _____   Phone _____

Address _____   City/St/Zip _____

Figure 9-1. Patient Registration Form.

DATE	PATIENT NO.	CHARGES	CREDITS	CUR. BALANCE	PREV BALANCE	NAME

PAID BY   ☐ CASH   ☐ VISA/MC   ☐ CHECK

OFFICE NEW PATIENT		UPPER EXTREMITY		NEW PATIENT-PT		STRAPPING	
99201	LEVEL 1	73000	CLAVICLE, COMPLETE	97799	EVAL-NEW PAT 30 MIN	29540	A4454 STRAP ANKLE
99202	LEVEL 2	71130	STERNOCLAV JNTS, COMP	00201	PT OFFICE VISIT-NC	29260	A4454 STRP ELB/WRIST
99203	LEVEL 3	73010	SCAPULA, COMPLETE	PROCEDURES		29280	A4454 HAND/FINGER
99204	LEVEL 4	73020	SHOULDER, 1V	64550	APPL OF TENS UNIT	29520	A4454 STRAP HIP
99205	LEVEL 5	73030	SHOULDER, 2V	97116	GAIT TRAINING	29530	A4454 STRAP KNEE
		193	SHOULDER, 3V ROUTINE	97124	MASSAGE	29240	A4454 STRAP SHOULDER
OFFICE ESTABLISHED PT		73050	AC JOINT, 2V	97250	MYOFAS REL/SOFT TIS MOB	29550	A4454 STRAP F0OT/TOES
99211	LEVEL 1	221	AC JOINT, BILAT 4V	97112	NEUROMUSCULAR RE-ED	MEDICAL SUPPLIES	
99212	LEVEL 2	73060	HUMEROUS, 2V	97530	THERAP ACTIV.-15 MIN	L4350	AIRCAST-STD
99213	LEVEL 3	73070	ELBOW, AP & LAT	97110	THERAP EXERC.-15 MIN	L4370	AIRCAST-LONG
99214	LEVEL 4	73080	ELBOW, COMP. 3V ROUTINE	97122	TRACTION-MANUAL	L4360	AC-WALK.BOOT
99215	LEVEL 5	73090	FOREARM, AP & LAT	MODALITIES		A4570(151)	AC TEN-ELB STRAP
200	POST OP/NC	73100	WRIST, AP & LAT	97032	ELECTRICAL STIM.-15 MIN	106	CAST SHOE
		73110	WRIST, 3V	97010	HOT PACK/COLD PACK	L3670	CLAVICLE STRAP
OFFICE OUTPATIENT CONSULTATION		218	WRIST, 5V ROUTINE	97033	IONTOPHORESIS - 15 MIN	L3914	CTR."RC" WRIST BR
99241	LEVEL 1	219	WRIST, 6V	97012	TRACTION - MECHANICAL	L3914(152)	CTR."RU" WRIST BR
99242	LEVEL 2	73120	HAND, 2V	97035	ULTRASOUND-15 MIN	E0112	CRUTCHES
99243	LEVEL 3	73130	HAND, MIN 3V	97016	VASOPNEUMATIC DEVICE	E0237	CRYOCUFF
99244	LEVEL 4	73140	FINGER, MIN 2V	97022	WHIRLPOOL	L3690(132)	DANEK AC IMMOB.
99245	LEVEL 5	BILATERAL				L1815	DJ HINGED KNEE BR
		156	X/R ANKLE 2 VW(AP/LAT)	TESTS & MEASUREMENTS		A4565	FASHION SLING
CONFIRMATORY CONSULTATION		157	X/R ANKLE 3VW	97750	PHYS. PERF TEST-15 MIN	L3040	FOOT ARCH SPPT
99271	LEVEL 1	160	X/R CALC. 2 VW	95851	KT 1000	E1399(254)	GEL ANTI-VIB GLOVE
99272	LEVEL 2	162	X/R ELBOW 2 VW	20950(101)	C. P. TEST MULT/BILAT	E1399(187)	HAND EXER. AID
99273	LEVEL 3	163	X/R ELBOW 3 VW	20950	C. P. TEST-SINGLE	L1830	KNEE IMMOBILIZER
99274	LEVEL 4	169	X/R FEMUR 2 VW	20950(100)	C. P. TEST-MULTI OR BILAT.	E1399(284)	LIONS PAW
99275	LEVEL 5	133	X/R FOOT 1 VW LAT	CASTS		L3020	LANGER ORTHO.
		159	X/R FOOT 3 VW	29065	LONG ARM	E1399(111)	LUMBAR/CERV ROLL
X-RAY SPINE & PELVIS		276	X/R FOOT AP'LAT 2 VW	29075	SHORT ARM	L0515	LUMBO/SAC SUPPT.
72010	ENTIRE, AP & LAT	164	X/R FOREARM 2 VW	29085	HAND TO LOWER ARM	L4210	ORTHO. REFURBISH
72020	SPINE, 1V	168	X/R HAND 3 VW	29345	LONG LEG	E1399(179)	PRO CALF SLEEVE
72040	CERVICAL, AP & LAT	167	X/R HAND 2 VW	29365	CYLINDER CAST	L1800(226)	PRO DR. M KNEE BR
72050	CERVICAL, 4V	161	X/R HUMERUS 2 VW	29405	SHORT LEG	L1800	PRO DR.MU BRACE
72052	CERVICAL, COMPLETE, 6V	155	X/R TIB & FIB 2 VW	29425	SHORT LEG-WALKING	A4570	PRO ELBOW SLEEVE
72070	THORACIC, AP & LAT	165	X/R WRIST 2 VW(AP/LAT)	29700	CAST REMOVAL/BIVALVING	L3710	PRO ELB HNGED BR
72080	THORACOLUMBAR SPINE,	166	X/R WRIST 3 VW	29085	THUMB CAST	L8190	PRO EXER. TRUNK
72100	LUMBOSACRAL, AP & LAT	170	X/R KNEE 3 VW OR LESS	SPLINTS		L1810	PRO HNG KNEE BR
72110	LUMBOSACRAL, 4V	170	X/R KNEE 4 VW OR MORE	29130	A4570 FINGER SPLINT	L1800(110)	PRO KNEE SLEEVE
72170	PELVIS, AP ONLY	278	COMP PRESS ACUTE	29125(249)	A4570 HAND BASED SPLT	L1825	PRO OSGOOD STRP
73520	PELVIS W/LAT HIP	277	X/R SHLDR 3 VW OR LESS	29105	A4570 LONG ARM SPLINT	E1399(115)	PRO THIGH SLVE.
72220	SACRUM & COCCYX 2V	221	X/R AC JNT 4 VW OR MORE	29125	A4570 SHORT ARM SPLINT	L3650(233)	SHOULDER PULLEY
72200	SACROILIAC JOINTS	224	X/R STANDING LEG BIL	29125(259)	A4570 SHORT ARM SPL(PC)	L3650(150)	SHOULDER IMMOB.
72190	PELVIS COMP 3V	286	X/R KNEE 4V ORBIT	29515	A4570 SHORT LEG SPLINT	L3650(245)	SHLD'R REHAB. KIT
LOWER EXTREMITY		MISCELLANEOUS		29126(257)	A4570 DYN. PRO SPLNT SUP	L3960	SHLD'R SUBL INHIB.
73500	HIP, UNILAT, 1V	71010	CHEST, 1V	29126	A4570 LARGE DYN. SPLINT	L3660	SHLD'R SAWA BR.
73510	HIP, COMP. 2V	71020	CHEST, 2V	29131(186)	A4570 SAFETY PIN SPLINT	L1960	SWEDO ANKLE BR.
73550	FEMUR, AP & LAT	71100	RIBS, 2V	29131	A4570 SMALL DYN. SPLINT		
73560	KNEE, 1V	71110	RIBS, BILAT	29105(275)	A4570 MUNSTER SPLINT		
73560	KNEE, AP & LAT	71120	STERNUM, 2V				
73562	KNEE, 3V	76499	X-RAY COPY				
73564	KNEE, 4V	76140	REVIEW OUTSIDE X-RAY				
73590	TIBIA & FIBULA, AP & LAT	93000	EKG				
73600	ANKLE, AP & LAT						
73610	ANKLE, COMP 3V						
73650	CALCANEUS, MIN 2V	INJECTION ASPIRATION					
73660	TOES MIN 2V	20600	SMALL JOINT				
73062	STANDING LEG	20605	INTERMEDIATE JOINT				
73620	FOOT AP & LAT	20610	LARGE JOINT				
73630	FOOT COMP 3V						

NEXT APPT.	DAY	DATE	TIME	CODE
Dr.				
PT				
DIAG.			DOI	

Figure 9-2. Patient Encounter Form.

diagnosis code must be included. These forms are generally customized to the medical practice and include the most common procedures that are routinely carried out by the practitioners as well as a listing of the most common diagnoses. It is important that the form contain written procedure and diagnosis codes as well as the corresponding numerical values. Having both of these available will make it much easier for data entry of the charges if the facility has a computerized billing system. Patients will often submit the claim directly to the insurance company themselves. In this situation, it is imperative that the form contain this information so that the patient will be reimbursed for services.

Step 2: Post Charges to the Daily Journal

Following each patient's visit to the health care facility, office personnel will record all charges to a daily record known as the accounts receivable journal or day sheet. This is a chronological summary of all of the charges that are posted to patient accounts on any given day and reflects an accurate accounting of charges, payments at the time of service, and total accounts receivable for the practice.

Step 3: Post Charges to Individual Patient Accounts

After recording charges to the daily accounts receivable journal, it then is necessary to post the charges to each patient's individual account. This account is considered a permanent record of the financial relationship that the patient has with the medical practice. Postings to the account must include date of service, detailed listing of all procedures and corresponding procedure code with accurate pricing, diagnosis code or codes, as well as any payments that were received from the patient at the time of the visit.

Step 4: Complete Insurance Claim Form

With all of the above information now available, it is then possible to complete an insurance claim form to be submitted to the insurance company or managed care organization for third party reimbursement. The standard Form HCFA-1500 (Figure 9-3) is accepted by most carriers. Blue Cross/Blue Shield requires the Form UB-92 (Figure 9-4) when submitting claims for rehabilitative services and durable medical equipment. When submitting a claim it is necessary that it be completed in detail. Information obtained from the new patient registration form to be included on the claim includes name, address, insurance company name, and account number. Specific medical procedures, procedural and diagnostic codes, and date of service information can be obtained from each individual patient account. Many of the medical software packages available today will pull together information from the patient registration screen, account postings, and insurance screen to automatically print insurance forms on a regular billing cycle. Once the insurance form is completed, it must be checked for accuracy with additional documentation attached including such information as letters of medical necessity for durable medical equipment. The patient's account will reflect that the form has been completed and sent to the insurance company for processing.[16,17]

ROLE OF THE NATIONAL ATHLETIC TRAINERS' ASSOCIATION IN THIRD PARTY REIMBURSEMENT

With a clear understanding of the history of health care reimbursement, ongoing changes within the system and the specific details of insurance reimbursement, it then

PLEASE
DO NOT
STAPLE
IN THIS
AREA

CARRIER →

HEALTH INSURANCE CLAIM FORM

PICA

1. MEDICARE   MEDICAID   CHAMPUS   CHAMPVA   GROUP HEALTH PLAN   FECA BLK LUNG   OTHER   1a. INSURED'S I.D. NUMBER   (FOR PROGRAM IN ITEM 1)
   (Medicare #)   (Medicaid #)   (Sponsor's SSN)   (VA File #)   (SSN or ID)   (SSN)   (ID)

2. PATIENT'S NAME (Last Name, First Name, Middle Initial)

3. PATIENT'S BIRTH DATE   MM   DD   YY   SEX   M   F

4. INSURED'S NAME (Last Name, First Name, Middle Initial)

5. PATIENT'S ADDRESS (No., Street)

6. PATIENT RELATIONSHIP TO INSURED   Self   Spouse   Child   Other

7. INSURED'S ADDRESS (No., Street)

CITY   STATE

8. PATIENT STATUS   Single   Married   Other   Employed   Full-Time Student   Part-Time Student

CITY   STATE

ZIP CODE   TELEPHONE (Include Area Code)   (   )

ZIP CODE   TELEPHONE (INCLUDE AREA CODE)   (   )

9. OTHER INSURED'S NAME (Last Name, First Name, Middle Initial)

10. IS PATIENT'S CONDITION RELATED TO:

11. INSURED'S POLICY GROUP OR FECA NUMBER

a. OTHER INSURED'S POLICY OR GROUP NUMBER

a. EMPLOYMENT? (CURRENT OR PREVIOUS)   YES   NO

a. INSURED'S DATE OF BIRTH   MM   DD   YY   SEX   M   F

b. OTHER INSURED'S DATE OF BIRTH   MM   DD   YY   SEX   M   F

b. AUTO ACCIDENT?   PLACE (State)   YES   NO

b. EMPLOYER'S NAME OR SCHOOL NAME

c. EMPLOYER'S NAME OR SCHOOL NAME

c. OTHER ACCIDENT?   YES   NO

c. INSURANCE PLAN NAME OR PROGRAM NAME

d. INSURANCE PLAN NAME OR PROGRAM NAME

10d. RESERVED FOR LOCAL USE

d. IS THERE ANOTHER HEALTH BENEFIT PLAN?   YES   NO   If yes, return to and complete item 9 a-d.

READ BACK OF FORM BEFORE COMPLETING & SIGNING THIS FORM.

12. PATIENT'S OR AUTHORIZED PERSON'S SIGNATURE I authorize the release of any medical or other information necessary to process this claim. I also request payment of government benefits either to myself or to the party who accepts assignment below.

SIGNED _____   DATE _____

13. INSURED'S OR AUTHORIZED PERSON'S SIGNATURE I authorize payment of medical benefits to the undersigned physician or supplier for services described below.

SIGNED _____

14. DATE OF CURRENT: ILLNESS (First symptom) OR INJURY (Accident) OR PREGNANCY (LMP)   MM   DD   YY

15. IF PATIENT HAS HAD SAME OR SIMILAR ILLNESS. GIVE FIRST DATE   MM   DD   YY

16. DATES PATIENT UNABLE TO WORK IN CURRENT OCCUPATION   MM   DD   YY   FROM   TO   MM   DD   YY

17. NAME OF REFERRING PHYSICIAN OR OTHER SOURCE

17a. I.D. NUMBER OF REFERRING PHYSICIAN

18. HOSPITALIZATION DATES RELATED TO CURRENT SERVICES   MM   DD   YY   FROM   TO   MM   DD   YY

19. RESERVED FOR LOCAL USE

20. OUTSIDE LAB?   YES   NO $ CHARGES

21. DIAGNOSIS OR NATURE OF ILLNESS OR INJURY. (RELATE ITEMS 1,2,3 OR 4 TO ITEM 24E BY LINE)

1. _____   3. _____
2. _____   4. _____

22. MEDICAID RESUBMISSION CODE   ORIGINAL REF. NO.

23. PRIOR AUTHORIZATION NUMBER

24. A DATE(S) OF SERVICE			B Place of Service	C Type of Service	D PROCEDURES, SERVICES, OR SUPPLIES (Explain Unusual Circumstances) CPT/HCPCS MODIFIER	E DIAGNOSIS CODE	F $ CHARGES	G DAYS OR UNITS	H EPSDT Family Plan	I EMG	J COB	K RESERVED FOR LOCAL USE
From MM DD YY	To MM DD YY											
1												
2												
3												
4												
5												
6												

25. FEDERAL TAX I.D. NUMBER   SSN   EIN

26. PATIENT'S ACCOUNT NO.

27. ACCEPT ASSIGNMENT? (For govt. claims see back)   YES   NO

28. TOTAL CHARGE $

29. AMOUNT PAID $

30. BALANCE DUE $

31. SIGNATURE OF PHYSICIAN OR SUPPLIER INCLUDING DEGREES OR CREDENTIALS (I certify that the statements on the reverse apply to this bill and are made a part thereof.)

SIGNED _____   DATE _____

32. NAME AND ADDRESS OF FACILITY WHERE SERVICES WERE RENDERED (If other than home or office)

33. PHYSICIAN'S, SUPPLIER'S BILLING NAME, ADDRESS, ZIP CODE & PHONE #

PIN#   GRP#

(APPROVED BY **AMA** COUNCIL ON MEDICAL SERVICE 8/88)   **PLEASE PRINT OR TYPE**   APPROVED OMB-0938-0008 FORM HCFA-1500 (12-90), FORM RRB-1500, APPROVED OMB-1215-0055 FORM OWCP-1500, APPROVED OMB-0720-0001 (CHAMPUS)

PATIENT AND INSURED INFORMATION

PHYSICIAN OR SUPPLIER INFORMATION

Figure 9-3. Form HCFA-1500.

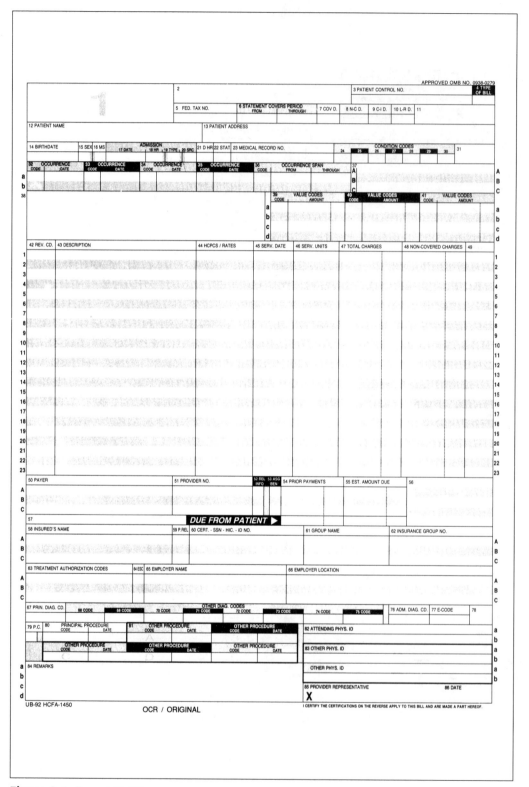

Figure 9-4. Form UB-92.

becomes important to review the internal and external environment as it relates to provider reimbursement. The National Athletic Trainers' Association (NATA) has been keeping a close watch on the changing national health care system. In 1995, the NATA set up the Reimbursement Advisory Group (RAG) to investigate managed care issues and plan strategies to help ensure that certified athletic trainers have a secure place in the evolving health care environment. A 3-year project (1996–1999) funded by the NATA Board of Directors through a grant to the NATA Research and Education Foundation was initiated with the formation of the RAG. The three primary goals of the group include: 1) education of athletic trainers on the issue of reimbursement, 2) development of a model approach to third-party payers for reimbursement of athletic training services, and 3) design and implementation of a clinical outcomes data study.[18]

Education of athletic trainers on the issue of reimbursement has primarily involved written communication through NATA publications, district and state newsletters, and presentations at local and national meetings. Several athletic trainer organizations are leading the way in education by establishing reimbursement committees. The Indiana Athletic Trainers Association appointed a task force in 1994 to investigate the feasibility of third party reimbursement for services rendered by athletic trainers in the state. Many other states have formed similar committees.

In addition to keeping members informed regarding the status of their work, these local committees are working closely with the NATA to lay the ground work for all reimbursement efforts on behalf of athletic trainers. NATA legal counsel has been involved in pursuing the appropriateness of contacting the insurance commissioners in each state to determine individual state insurance regulations.

In conjunction with the RAG, the Indiana Reimbursement Committee initiated meetings with managed care networks, self-insured employer groups, and workers' compensation payers in an effort to better understand the perspective of third-party payers. Reimbursement committees in Massachusetts, Missouri, Ohio, and Washington are also working closely with the RAG to educate third-party payers in their state about the role and responsibilities of athletic trainers.

A model approach is being developed by the RAG for use by these state committees. The core information in this model includes athletic training competencies, organizational membership issues, Board of Certification credentialing information, American Medical Association endorsement of the profession, requirements for accreditation of educational programs, and outcomes data. This information will be made available to state reimbursement committees. It will be the responsibility of the individual state committees to insert information regarding state athletic training regulatory acts and legal interpretations of statutes. Each state will also receive information regarding the use of the packets in approaching third-party payers.

In order for health care providers to secure a place in the national health care system, they must be able to demonstrate the effects of their intervention on the patient's health status. Athletic trainers are no exception. The development of support data, which measures the results of intervention, is known as outcomes research. Many managed care payers are now requiring outcomes studies when evaluating a contract.

In 1995, the NATA came to the forefront of allied health care organizations in initiating and developing an outcomes research instrument specific to the profession of athletic training. The focus of the national outcomes research project is on functional outcomes.

This includes a measure of the patient's physical, mental, and social well-being, as well as the patient's perception of function and overall satisfaction. Cost-effectiveness will also be addressed in terms of early intervention, time lost from activity, and number of treatment visits within a certain time period.[19]

An outcomes vendor was selected by the RAG subcommittee in 1995. BIO*Analysis Systems from Denver, Colorado was selected to develop, validate, and conduct the NATA outcomes study.[20] Lyle Knudson, president of BIO*Analysis and former coach, worked to develop a tool specifically geared toward athletic training rather than simply adapting a pre-existing tool from other associated professions (see Chapter 20).

Following preliminary field testing and refinement, the Athletic Training Outcomes Assessment instrument was validated in late 1995. Representative data are currently being collected at more than 100 athletic training sites around the country. These sites include high school, college, clinical and industrial settings. The one-page form is designed to provide a comprehensive definition of outcomes. It requires that both the athletic trainer and the patient respond on a scale of 0 (critical problem) to 4 (no problem) to questions about general health and functional abilities.[20]

SUMMARY

This is a critical time in our nation's health care history. It is imperative that providers have a clear understanding of the ever-changing environment in which they are working. The role of a health care provider must be clearly defined with accurate documentation of clinical outcomes that are achieved in providing consumer services.

Study Questions

1. What two entitlement programs were established as part of the Social Security Act of 1965?
2. List the four primary sources of reimbursement for health care services.
3. What factors prompted the significant changes in the American health care system?
4. Describe the prospective payment system.
5. List the principle constructs of the managed care model and describe how the system works.
6. What are the five types of insurance plans?
7. What classification systems should be used in reporting clinical diagnoses and procedures?
8. Describe the five-step process of submitting an insurance claim.
9. What are the three goals of the NATA Reimbursement Advisory Group?
10. What professional information should a health care provider attempt to convey when approaching third-party payers about reimbursement for services?

References

1. Nosse LJ, Friberg DG. *Management Principles for Physical Therapists.* Baltimore, Md: Williams & Wilkins; 1992:1-17.

2. Norbeck TB. Rising health care costs: Telling the truth. *Conn Med.* 1990;54:142-146.

3. Rheinecker P. Catholic healthcare enters a new world. *Health Prog.* 1990;31-36.

4. Horting M. HMOs and the physical therapist: A growing relationship. *Clin Management.* 1987;7:30-35.

5. Kiesler LA, Morton TL. Psychology and public policy in the "health care revolution." *Am Psychology.* 1988;43:993-1003.

6. Berk PD. Restructuring American health care financing: First of all do no harm. *Hepatology.* 1993;18:206-215.

7. Daschle TA, Cohen RJ, Rice CL. Health care reform. *Am Psychol.* 1993;48:265-269.

8. Dowd B, Christianson J, Feldman R, Wisner C, Klein J. Issues regarding health plan payments under Medicare and recommendations for reform. *Milbank Q.* 1992;70:423-453.

9. Dore D. Effect of the Medicare prospective payment system on the utilization of physical therapy. *Physical Therapy.* 1987;67: 964-966.

10. Kerrey B, Hofshire PJ. Hidden problems in current health care financing and potential changes. *Am Pschol.* 1993;261:261-264.

11. Bender D, Leone B, eds. *Health care in America.* San Diego, Calif: Greenhaven Publishers, Inc.; 1994.

12. Reed SK, Hennessy K, Brown SW, Fray J. Capitation from a provider's perspective. *Hospital & Community Psychiatry.* 1992;43:1173-1175.

13. Benjamin K. Outcomes research and the allied health professional. *J Allied Health.* 1995;24:3-12.

14. Harada N, Sofaer S, Kominski G. Functional status outcomes in rehabilitation: Implications for prospective payment. *Medical Care.* 1993;31:345-357.

15. Nosse LJ, Friberg DG. *Management Principles for Physical Therapists.* Baltimore, Md: Williams & Wilkins; 1992:27-140.

16. Beck, DF. *Principles of Reimbursement in Health Care.* Rockville, Md.: Aspen Publishers; 1984.

17. Rowell JC, ed. *Understanding Medical Insurance: A Step-by-Step Guide.* Albany, NY: Delmar Publishers;1994.

18. Campbell D. Workshop on third party reimbursement. *NATA News.* 1996;34.

19. Webster K. Outcomes research in health care. *NATA News.* 1995;26.

20. Webster K. Outcomes research project update. *NATA News.* 1996;14.

Suggested Readings

Bingaman J, Frank RG, Billy CL. Combining a global health budget with a market-driven delivery system. *Am Psychol.* 1993;48:270-276.

Franks P, Nutting PA, Clancy CM. Health care reform, primary care, and the need for research. *JAMA.* 1993;270:1449-1453.

Levit KR, Lazenby HC, Cowan CA, Letsch SW. Health care spending by state: New estimates for policy making. *Health Affairs.* 1993;7-25.

Menzel PT. Equality, autonomy, and efficiency: What health care system should we have? *J Med Philos.* 1992;17:33-57.

Nicoll LH, Niman NB. Deficit reduction and health care expenditures. *J Nurs Adm.* 1991;21:35-39.

Piascik P. Simple steps to reimbursement success. *American Pharmacy.* 1995;NS35:9-10.

Reinhardt UE, Madison J. Regulated fees or regulated competition? Implications for young physicians. *JAMA*. 1993;269:1713-1714.

Schramm CJ. Economics. *JAMA*. 1993;263:2635-2637.

Siu AL. Conflicting aims. Voluntary health insurance and contemporary medical practice. *Arch Intern Med*. 1993;153:457-463.

Stewart DL, Abein SH, eds. *Documenting Functional Outcomes in Physical Therapy*. St. Louis, Mo: Mosby, 1993.

Uili RM, Wood R. The effect of third-party payers on the clinical decision making of physical therapists. *Soc Sci Med*. 1995;40:873-879.

Volpp K. Costs, benefits and the changing ethos of medicine (editorial). *JAMA*. 1993;269:1712-1714.

Welk FJ. Reimbursement for physical therapists: Facing the challenge of the future. *Ortho Physical Ther Clin of North Am*. 1993;2:367-374.

Acknowledgments

Special thanks to Kathy Malone, MA, ATC, for her assistance in gathering information relating to athletic trainer reimbursement.

Clinical Marketing

Jim Clover, MEd, ATC, PTA

OBJECTIVES

Upon completion of this chapter, the student will be able to accomplish the following:

1. Understand the strategic planning process, the decision-making process, and how they work together with internal and external environment assessment

2. Identify different methods of record keeping for referrals and recognize their effect on marketing strategies

3. Assess the mix of product, price, place, promotion, people, and pride

4. Evaluate the strengths and weaknesses of different types of advertising methods

5. Position and preserve market segments

6. Evaluate the benefits of each marketing segment and make necessary changes

7. Establish a marketing philosophy that will be best suited for a particular environment

8. Use hints and myths for practical use

9. Interpret myths in marketing

The best marketing scheme ever may belong to the person who sold the idea, or maybe just the product, that drive-thru automatic transaction machines at banks needed to have Braille. Think about it.

Athletic trainers, sports medicine providers, and caregivers need to "talk the talk" to get the appropriate people to listen to what they have to say. Athletic trainers must sell themselves and their product, and be able to define "sports medicine" as a multispecialty approach that can solve most health related problems with an efficient solution.

Name recognition is a problem, without question, for the certified athletic trainer. Many years ago, athletic trainers were known as horse trainers. Now, many are known as personal fitness trainers. Essentially, that leaves an individual with three options: be a horse trainer, be a personal trainer, or educate an audience on what a Certified Athletic Trainer does. Who and what is a Certified Athletic Trainer?

To better understand the marketing of a profession, some basic definitions need to be addressed:

- *Marketing*: Process of planning and executing the conception, pricing, promotion, and distribution of ideas, goods, services, organizations, and events to *create exchanges* that satisfy individual and organizational objectives.
- *Advertising:* Paid, nonpersonal communications by business firms, nonprofit organizations and individuals who are identified in their advertising message and who you hope to inform or persuade the members of a particular audience.
- *Promotion:* Function of informing, persuading, and influencing the buyer's purchase decision.

THE STRATEGIC PLANNING PROCESS

The strategic planning process is a method in which an individual can organize and evaluate his or her project by pulling together staff and others in the area with similar interest in the project. The strategic plan accomplishes the following:

1. Forces setting of objectives
2. Clarifies opportunities and threats
3. Defines target markets and appropriate strategies
4. Focuses attention on key issues that will determine project success
5. Establishes a framework for making decisions
6. Provides a basis for measuring performance

For the athletic trainer, the development and implementation of a *strategic plan* is done somewhat like a treatment plan. Just as the athletic trainer's treatment plan serves the needs of the athlete or patient, strategic planning matches the characteristics and needs of potential consumers and/or referral sources in an organized method. This is considered a *marketing orientation* as opposed to a *product orientation*; it means the athletic trainer is responding to those who need and will use their planned services or product. These would be future patients or insurance carriers that determine the providers for the patients.

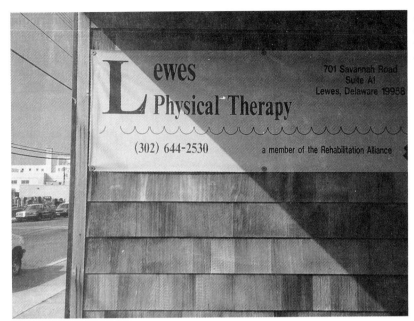

Figure 10-1. An example of a logo used to identify this particular clinical facility.

ELEMENTS FOR THE STRATEGIC PLANNING PROCESS

The following considerations should be assessed when a strategic plan is developed:
1. Name of event or project to be established
2. The strategic planning team (made up from the idea people)
3. The decision-making team ("players," money, and influential people)
4. Internal and external environmental assessment
5. Market segmentation
6. Macro objectives
7. Strategies and goals
8. The marketing mix
9. Positioning
10. Plan finalization and review
11. Evaluation of short-term and long-term goals

Name of Event or Project

The clinical owner should always make an attempt to connect the name of the facility with the type of product or service provided when marketing the facility. This process may be enhanced by developing a logo and standard colors that will set the facility apart from others and create an individualized image. When doing this, it would be a wise investment for the owner to protect the facility's identity through a trademark or any other method that would establish a form of ownership (Figure 10-1).

The Strategic Planning Team

The strategic planning team can be made up of anyone the owner deems necessary to make this plan pull together and come into fruition. He or she can search for and evaluate people in his or her area who may be interested in the outcome of the business, if in some way that will also benefit that person (i.e., win-win). To put together an outreach program, a clinical owner might enlist the superintendent of the schools, a board member, a football coach, a female coach, as well as key people from his or her medical group. This may also help to solidify the concept being promoted to the rest of the group and give them ownership in the project. Personnel from the medical group might include any of the following people:

- Medical director
- Referred specialists from the medical staff
- Physical therapist
- Certified athletic trainer
- Marketing specialist
- Administrator
- Financial service provider
- Patient services

The Decision-Making Team

The decision-making team has the potential to become very time-consuming because of a multidisciplinary team involvement. Once the general concept is agreed upon it is highly recommended that daily decisions and the initiation of new ideas be made by no more than two competent people, one from the strategic planning team and one from the decision-making team. All key members will approach the situation from a different perspective and with a different set of concerns, but it is essential for them to keep the following points in mind and focus on answering questions that will meet the main objective:

1. Why is the service being offered?
2. To whom will the service be provided?
3. Through whom will patients/athletes be referred?
4. What unmet need exists?
5. What is the reimbursement source?
6. How will availability of the service be communicated?
7. Who will provide the service?
8. Where will it be provided, and when?
9. What is the time frame for the evaluation/assessment of the primary objectives?
10. How will it be financed?
11. How long will it take for this program to meet each objective?
12. How will you know if you are successful?

In order for a plan or program to meet the objectives, everyone needs to understand that not everyone will be satisfied with every part of the plan. However, the majority must carry the project so the process can move to the next step. Accountability must be built into the plan that describes deadlines and expectations. When the final decision is made, the entire committee must stand behind the plan. Underfunding, understaffing, and underpromoting have resulted in more project failures than desirable.

Internal Environment Assessment

Internal environment assessment involves the analyzing and defining of the factors *within* the organization that may help or hinder the development and growth of a program or service. The following are factors to be considered:

- Organization's strengths, weaknesses, and reputation
- Existing services and how they will help or hinder a program
- Staff capabilities (e.g., what qualifications, skills, motivation do they have in this project? [ownership])
- Location and space (location/location/location)
- Access of service (e.g., reimbursement, convenience, transportation, hours of operations)
- Competitive factors (e.g., Who can refer from within? Does someone else in the organization already have something similar going on?)
- Developmental capital (e.g., staff, equipment, promotion)
- Commitment (e.g., support must come from administration, rehabilitation, marketing, and key players)

External Environment Assessment

A clinical owner should pay careful attention in providing a clear picture of the external opportunities, threats, and constraints that may have an impact on the intended program or services. This includes competitors, market characteristics, and consumer wants and needs. The assessment should identify current and future elements that may influence the how, when, and where of the programs implemented. Special considerations might include gathering demographic data with respect to the community and surrounding areas, major employers, third-party payers, local health plans, and their requirements and restrictions on outpatient rehabilitation. All influential items should be part of the assessment. Table 10-1 displays a list of influential items to be considered.

Referral Physician Survey

It is beneficial for an athletic trainer to find out what a physician's practice does in relation to the service he or she can provide, and how the athletic trainer might be able to improve that service. One trick is to set up a referral source data bank to understand how the marketing process is working. This will also establish the market segment the clinical owner should concentrate on, and the part that may now be reachable under the current conditions.

Table 10-1

Influential Items that Should Be Included During an External Environmental Assessment for Marketing

1. Population size
2. Household size and make-up
3. Growth projections
4. Age distribution
5. Income distribution
6. Education levels
7. Occupation (blue collar/white collar)
8. Ethnic or cultural make-up
9. Behavior patterns
10. Leisure activities
11. Employers
12. Junior high schools
13. High schools in the area
14. Colleges and universities in the area
15. Professional athletic teams in the area
16. Amateur and club teams in the area
17. Employment/job growth

Health Care Trends

Once clinical owners have evaluated the external environment, they should look at what is going on in other communities with programs similar to theirs. National magazines and journals are great resources to help keep abreast of other opportunities in the area. Networking with other professionals outside the area is also a great way to share ideas and opportunities; for example, if an athletic trainer needs to find extended rehabilitation services for a patient when an insurer decides to stop payments.

Potential Referral Sources

When evaluating potential referral sources look at every possible source. It is the athletic trainer's responsibility to ensure that his or her program meets the needs of the potential sources. As the old saying goes, "If you don't take care of the customers, someone else will." An example of places to look for potential referral sources might include the following:

- High school athletes, college athletes
- Family and friends of high school athletes, college athletes
- Family practice patients
- Members of athletic clubs
- Employees of major businesses in town
- Service group participants (Chamber of Commerce)

Competition

It is important for clinical owners to know who else in the marketplace is offering similar services, where they are located, what services they provide, when they are available, and at what cost. This can be done in a number of ways. There is nothing wrong or unethical about investigating the ways in which a competitor operates. In fact, it is vital to the success of any business. Reviewing the promotional and educational information that other providers use to market is an easy place to start. Learning as much as possible about a competitor can place any company in a competitive position.

Reimbursement Potential

It is important for new owners to find out the potential for reimbursement, either from insurance or self-pay. Workers' compensation, private insurance, and HMOs should be evaluated. Income projections allow for a realistic view of the viability of the services that are being considered. Efforts should be made to identify similar programs with which to compare, whether they are in the facility's area or not, and information should be used to network for better outcomes through the facility's services. Then market those outcomes.

Market Segmentation

Market segmentation is the process of dividing the market into groups of potential customers with common needs, values, or ability to pay. Clinical owners must determine the extent to which they will compete without being at risk of losing any possible referral sources that are already established. When assessing a segmented market, there are a number of places an individual can look to for potential customers. The list of choices is essentially infinite, but will depend upon whether or not the owner does his or her homework (Table 10-2).

Table 10-2
List of Potential Customers in a Segmented Market

- Other physicians
- Schools at all levels
- Other therapist and rehabilitation programs
- Patients
- Families
- Insurance companies
- Health plans (HMOs, PPOs)

- Chiropractors
- Health clubs
- Adult athletic leagues
- Private athletic clubs (dance, gymnastics)
- Dentists
- Podiatrists
- Youth sports

Macro Objectives

Macro objectives include a planning process to establish broad, overall objectives to set performance targets and measure progress. For example, a sports medicine program may have a macro objective to break even financially by the second year. In order to meet macro objectives, definitive terms must be established. Using the previous example, a clinical owner would need to know the financial numbers that are involved to break even.

Strategies and Goals

Strategies are a broad initiative designed to provide a **measurable** means of achieving macro objectives. For example, a macro objective of potential referrals can be established, but to do so, referral needs to be defined.

Referral Breakdown

1. Direct—the patients whom the trainer walks in directly
2. Indirect—the patients whom the trainer sends to their primary care physician (PCP) and they send back
3. Name recognition—the patients heard or saw the name
4. Phone book
5. Other marketing endeavors (e.g., radio advertising, program advertising)

Method for Tracking Referrals

1. Every patient seen must fill out the minimal information to be accessible for cross reference and evaluation of the marketing system and plan. Tracking referrals may seem to be tedious at times, but every attempt should be made to make this one of the foundations of a marketing plan. Referral tracking can either make or break a practice.
2. Every patient arrives at a clinic some way—there may be a minimal percentage of patients that have no referral source. However, if there is a large number of patients without good referral information, the system does not work and the program evaluation will suffer.
3. Registration questionnaires provide an opportunity to retain information such as geographic demographics from the patient population.
4. The receptionist must take ownership in the referral tracking system and the patient compliance in making their scheduled appointments.
5. The referral information must be attainable; that is, capable of being accessed in a reasonable time for timely evaluation of the marketing plan.

Strategic goals must be SMART:

- Specific
- Measurable
- Attainable
- Relevant
- Traceable

Strategic goals are critical in allowing goals of evaluation to be met in a reasonable time frame. Time frames can be anywhere from 6-month to 3-year intervals, and are important to assess because they may reveal trends that are occurring in the facility or community.

The Marketing Mix

The basic foundation that forms the marketing mix involves the four "Ps": Product, Price, Place, and Promotion. However, with the market the way it is, there is no reason why patient relations, positioning, and pride in what is being done (from the maintenance man who fixes the light bulb to the physician who treats the patients) could not be considered.

Product

By its very nature, a sports medicine facility may be expected to possess the most modern equipment, have access to the latest supplies, and employ a friendly, knowledgeable, outgoing staff to appeal to its clients. The entire staff, from the receptionist to the maintenance person, must take ownership in the product for the consumer to really believe the sincerity of the product.

The product must work on all levels when in the eyes of the consumer. All aspects should be considered important: the way the building looks, the colors that are used, how the people look, the background music—everything must be clean and present with a fresh aroma. Consumers have a sense of smell, sight, touch, and sound and they will use them. Therefore, the clinical owner should take advantage of his or her senses. Large businesses use these senses (e.g., Disney World). Without question they do a great job. Their efforts are very noticeable, and it is obvious that all of the employees take pride in their appearance and demeanor.

Price

The price of the product refers to the actual cost of the service. A critical component involves understanding what is a reasonable allowable markup. It also involves looking into the alternative payment options, such as cash or payment plans for when the insurance stops paying following a given number of treatments. An owner may decide to submit insurance for his or her clients, or give them information about their insurance. If they are unhappy with their options, the clinical owner may be in a position to give them a suitable alternative. The bottom line is to meet the market sector.

The perception of value created by nonfinancial factors, such as being the educational source for sports medicine, being the service of choice for all the athletes in the area, and being seen as the sports medicine coverage group for all the athletic events in your area, is important, too. Soft cost when pricing items should be added. This means if the clinic provides first aid coverage for a road race and the event does not have money to pay for

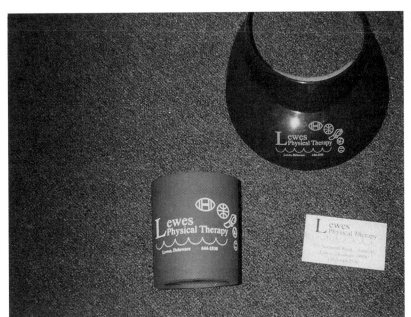

Figure 10-2. Examples of promoting a facility using everyday products.

the services, a true cost for the services rendered can be determined. Once this is established, this cost can be turned into a trade for advertising space and marketing opportunities.

Place

Place refers to the location in which the service is provided, as well as any mobile opportunities that the clinical owner establishes. The place in an outreach program may vary; it is wherever the services are being rendered. For example, if a trainee is working the county wrestling tournament and providing the first aid, he or she should advertise by hanging banners and wearing clothes that clearly identify his or her affiliation. A representative from a clinic cannot be every place at once, but if a rotational schedule is developed, the clinic will be able to make worthwhile communication with the area contacts (e.g., schools). A single location in a large geographic area can be a problem for patients needing treatment with any type of regularity. The schedule has to meet the needs of the patients. For example, the clinic might be open for the athletes from 6:00 AM until 8:00 AM and 12:00 Noon until 1:00 PM, Monday through Friday. These might be the slower times for the clinic. During the fall the clinic might be open on Saturdays after the football games for those athletes and athletes from other sports participating at that time (e.g., cross country, water polo). These hours should be established around school and practice schedules. Also, this schedule should allow the working parents time to bring the kids in without missing work.

Promotion/ Advertising

Promoting and advertising are the methods of communicating the message about the product or service to the purchasing public (Figure 10-2). This only happens after the product, the marketing mix, and the geographic market have all been defined. Table 10-3 lists some possible ideas and techniques that could be utilized as a source to promote and advertise. Although this list is extensive, by no means is it exhaustive. In addition, the strengths and weaknesses for some of these methods are examined in Table 10-4.

Table 10-3
Possible Ideas and Techniques to Promote and Advertise the Clinic

- Brochures
- Newsletter (some type of return information is very important to evaluate the readership of the newsletter)
- Educational pamphlets (e.g., what to do for a sprained ankle, how to access your medical group with the types of insurance that they can purchase)
- Direct mail (e.g., special educational programs coming up)
- Media exposure (e.g., well-written news releases of what the clinic is doing)
- Presentations to clients (e.g., physicians, coaches)
- Exhibits (e.g., health fairs, road races, sign-up time for health care sign-ups)
- Special service events (e.g., Chamber of Commerce, Junior League)
- Speaker's bureau (e.g., available to speak on sports medicine-related topics)
- Public education forums (e.g., bring in the trainers in the area and go over face mask removal using the Trainer's Angel, do a series on injury prevention for different sports, present a taping clinic)
- Phone book (advertisement should stand out in a crowded page, and found in all related parts of the phone book)
- Advertising for program/magazine/newspapers (e.g., information, return request)
- Television (e.g., cable)
- Radio (e.g., spot advertisement: "Snow report brought to you by ....")
- Signs—where and what type (e.g., ball parks)
- Education (e.g., high school, adult learning, college, first aid training)
- Sponsorship of teams, individuals, athletic events (watch for proper exposure)
- Participate in athletic events (e.g., corporate challenge, road races)
- Establish a tradition (e.g., All-Star Football Game, scholarship)
- Vehicle advertising (e.g., signs on a company van)
- Receptions for physicians
- Barbecues for coaches
- Equipment demonstrations (e.g., different types of knee braces, different types of shoulder pads)
- Member in athletic organizations ("Sports Medicine" consultant)
- Member of local athletic groups (e.g., Chamber of Commerce, athletic council)

Positioning

The process of positioning involves the creation of an image in the mind of the consumer or the referral source. The image should define the various entities that a clinic wishes to portray. What this simply means is establishing a reputation. Positioning also means a clinic being in the right place to receive maximum benefit for its services. It is essential that clinical owners obtain the insurance contracts and work with the major companies to control the patient's care.

Table 10-4
Strengths and Weaknesses of Advertisement and Promotional Approaches

Strengths	Weaknesses
Television (public or cable)	
High impact	High production cost
Audience selectivity	Uneven delivery by market
Schedule when needed	Upfront commitment required
Fast awareness	If not a local station, may have no impact on
Sponsorship available	area
Merchandising possible	
Must be local	
Radio	
Low cost per contact	Nonintrusive medium
Audience selectivity	Audience per spot small
Schedule when needed	No visual impact
Length can vary	High total cost for good reach
Personalities available	Clutter within spot market
Magazines	
Audience selectivity	Long lead time needed
Editorial association	Readership accumulates slowly
Long life	Uneven delivery by market
Large audience per insert	Cost premiums for regional or demographic
Excellent color	editions
Minimal waste	
Merchandising possible	
Newspaper	
Large audience	Difficult to target
Immediate reach	High waste
Short lead time	High cost national use
Market flexibility	Minimal positioning
Good upscale coverage	Clutter
Information advertising	
Poster, Billboards	
High reach	No depth of message
High frequency of exposure	High cost for national use
Minimal waste	Best positions already taken
Can localize	No audience selectivity
Flexible scheduling	Minimum 1 month purchase

Patient Relations

Patient relations can be the most cost-effective and most crucial element in the strategic planning process. It involves activities to ensure that the current customers and referral sources are satisfied with the services the clinic renders. This is an ongoing process and may include any of the following:

- Responding quickly to physicians
- Maintaining and improving skills as an athletic trainer
- Maintaining modern equipment
- Adapting a schedule that is for the patients
- Extending courtesy and compassion to the families
- Conducting discharge surveys
- Responding to patient and physician complaints
- Influencing waiting room conduct, giving the patients something to do while they wait (e.g., up-to-date magazines, not old torn up periodicals)

Be honest with patients if the doctor or someone else is running behind. It is the job of the receptionist to give patients honest information and suggest alternative activities to do while they wait or the option to come back at another time. Some groups even give their patients beepers if the doctor is running behind, so they could have the freedom to do other things they need to do. The patient's time is just as valuable as the trainer's time.

Plan Finalization and Review

Once the plan has been approved, the strategy team leader should remind everyone of their responsibilities. This group will evaluate progress, modify strategies, and coordinate activities. The main activity will be a review process. At some point in a strategic marketing plan, there must be a thorough review of the program's expected requirements and benefits. The expected income by source, operational expenses, and return to investors should be explored.

Evaluation

Is evaluation successful? A business owner needs only to compare objectives, strategies, and goals with actual results. This information should have both qualitative and quantitative data. An evaluation method should be set up from day one. It should be put in the system in a way that can be understood. The referral breakdown numbers should be examined. This includes those who came through direct and indirect means. It also includes those who came in because they heard of or saw the clinic's services advertised. This is important for the clinical owner to know because it gives him or her a sense of successful promotional efforts. Again, a tracking system needs to be in place so that every athlete who is seen must fill out the minimal information to be accessible in the main system for cross reference if he or she comes in at another time. It is difficult in a big practice to track everyone. Registration questionnaires and the gathering of information by the receptionist will aid in this process. Every patient arrived at the facility some way, and there should only be a minimal percentage of patients that have no referral source. If this number is large, then the system of tracking may not be working sufficiently. As a result, the evaluation of the program may be inadequate.

MARKETING PHILOSOPHY

Marketing is everyone's business. Satisfaction of the customers' wants and needs is the ultimate goal. To achieve this level, everyone in the organization must have ownership in the program. Unfortunately, many managers lose sight of customer needs because of stacks of paperwork and reports that require the time once designated for patient care. The importance of the telephone must be remembered. People in a health care system, in many cases, are in some form of discomfort and need help. The receptionist and anyone else taking outside calls must understand that the telephone is a business window to the outside world. Interaction is key, as it may be the first impression that is left with a client. A great impression must be made. If the insurance clerk trying to verify insurance coverage is rude, if documentation and reports are slow to reach the referring doctor or employer, and if the employers are kept on hold for long periods, the business will suffer as a result of negative interpersonal skills. People must be courteous, educated in their respected areas, and willing to bend over backwards to make sure that problems receive proper attention. All efforts to do so should be done without causing an inconvenience to the patient. Simply said, to succeed, a clinic must have a patient/athlete/customer-first attitude!

SUMMARY

With a strategic plan that clearly identifies the goals and objectives, an organization can chart the course it selects while meeting the needs of patients and the community it serves. An organization's services are valuable, and should be paid for everything. If the clinical owner has to work a bike race for free, then the clinic should be a sponsor. For example, many of the athletic trainers for the Olympics work for free and so there should be a trade off. All the time spent should be totaled and the NATA should receive that sponsorship reimbursement. If an athletic trainer is doing it for the clinic, a formula should be created that will determine trade off reimbursement rates. If there is more than one organization involved in an event, the sponsorship reimbursement can be given back to the NATA, district, or state organization. Outcome studies of marketing efforts are just as important as the actual advertisement or promotion itself. Beyond changes endangered by demographic trends and emerging technologies, the major issues that will shape the future of rehabilitation involve *changes in payment mechanisms*. The future of rehabilitation includes changes in payment mechanisms and the demand for cost accountability, the demand for performance documentation, changes in the competitive environment, and shortage of qualified rehabilitation professionals. If an athletic trainer cannot be accessed, he or she will eventually fail. Therefore a noteworthy part of any plan is for athletic trainers to be as accessible as possible and still provide good care. The demand for cost accountability is foremost. Opportunities in rehabilitation are increasing. There is a greater interest in returning injured employees and athletes to work and sports as soon as possible, and more concern about rehabilitation of the older athlete. The primary objective of strategic planning in outpatient rehabilitation is to develop and support a *lasting* competitive advantage. The essence of strategy formulation is coping with competition. One of the easiest ways to think of strategic planning is to contrast effectiveness (e.g., "Doing the right things") with efficiency (e.g., "Doing things right"). Strategic planning involves selecting the right things to do and to be. Services should be developed that meet the wants and needs of the specific customer group(s) for the program.

Marketing Myths

- *It is good to have a great deal of **white space** in advertisements, brochures, and other printed material.* Customers and prospects are not interested in white space. They are interested in information and services. The message should be interesting reading and worthy of the time they spent reading the information.
- *Sell the sizzle and not the steak.* The easiest way to sell a service is as the solution to a problem. Customers need to know an easy way to access the athletic trainer—show them the way.
- *Great marketing works instantly.* Great marketing is made up of creating a desire for what is being offered to the consumers. The time-delay factor of a marketing program must be considered.
- *Public relations stories have a short life span.* If a newspaper or magazine runs an article on an athletic trainer and his or her services, the trainer should make it last. The article can be framed and copies can be sent around to key people.
- *Quality is the main determination in influencing potential patients.* Quality is the second most important factor in influencing potential customers. Confidence and trust in service are the main determinant.
- *Money can be saved by producing marketing materials inside the company.* The way to view production of marketing materials is to recognize it as a place to protect the marketing investment. The brightest marketing strategy can be completely undone by a hint of unprofessionalism in brochures, advertisements, signs, letters, and so forth.
- *Once a solid customer base is established, marketing can be stopped.* It is possible to cut down on marketing but it should not be stopped. There are always new customers coming and going through a marketing segment.

Study Questions

1. Using the phone book's yellow pages, evaluate the advertisements for rehabilitative services.
2. If you were putting together a "Strategic Planning Process," what persons would you include?
3. How does the decision-making of the company process relate to the marketing outcome?
4. What are some of the key items that an athletic trainer would want a consumer to retain after leaving his or her establishment?
5. What would be the best type of marketing for a newly established athletic therapy business?
6. What would be some of the potential downfalls for any marketing program?

The Athletic Trainer as a Personnel Manager

Jeff G. Konin, MEd, ATC, MPT
Phillip B. Donley, MS, PT, ATC

OBJECTIVES

Upon completion of this chapter, the student will be able to accomplish the following:

1. Identify various managerial philosophies and styles and discuss their implications

2. Describe the four major functions of a manager

3. List the roles and responsibilities of a manager

4. Understand the keys to effective management of personnel

5. Explain the importance of employee performance evaluations and the steps one should take to design sound assessment programs

While the increase in the number of athletic trainers entering the clinical setting has been identified, it becomes apparent that many individuals will eventually take on managerial type roles in these settings. A number of currently existing facilities have already implemented titles such as "manager of athletic training services," "clinical administrator," or "coordinator of athletic training services." While the new graduate may not find him- or herself in these positions, he or she should not underestimate the rate of growth that athletic trainers are faced with today in the clinical setting, especially sports medicine clinics.

An interested student would be hard pressed to locate regularly offered continuing education that teaches athletic trainers personnel management skills. It can be hypothesized that the lack of educational opportunities in this area may be a result of two issues. The first, by their very nature, athletic trainers are good communicators and work well with people. Therefore, based on this assumption, courses that address issues such as managing people would not be very appealing to a professional who already considers this a professional strength.

Another reason for the lack of personnel management related coursework in athletic training education may be related to the history of the athletic trainer's role in the clinical setting. In most cases, the athletic trainer simply held a clinician type status. All personnel and administrative managerial responsibilities were left to those with expertise in the respected areas. One concern with this approach is that people who are managed by others that may not truly understand their educational training and job responsibility have some apprehensive feelings with respect to decision-making processes regarding athletic training.

The purposes of this chapter are to discuss the roles and responsibilities of personnel management and describe what are considered to be the essential components of effective managing. While these tools may serve to didactically prepare an athletic trainer for a managerial position in the clinical setting, it should be emphasized that each individual facility is unique in its own way, and that this information should not serve as a substitute for on-the-job training and experience.

DEFINITION OF MANAGEMENT

There is no single, universally accepted, standard definition of the word "management." For the purposes of this discussion, management can be defined as "that process by which managers create, direct, maintain, and operate purposive organizations through systematic, coordinated, and cooperative human effort."[1]

By defining management as a process, several key implications can be assumed. First, the dynamic nature of managing is indicated, in that no fixed or rigid formula is used. Second, management as a process can imply that activity actually occurs over varying spans of time. Third, it can be assumed that the process is ongoing, and that change is an ever-present reality. And fourth, the action set forth by managing has the potential to control to some level the nature, degree, extent, and pace of change within an organizational structure. Most importantly, it presents the opportunity to create an efficient, effective organization that is highly productive with strong morale.

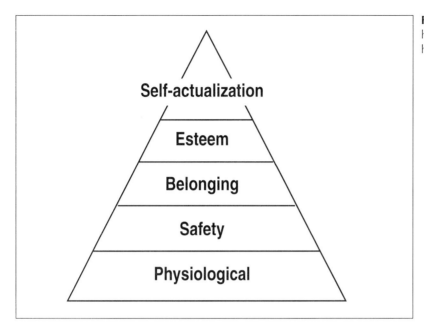

Figure 11-1. Maslow's hierarchical approach to human needs.

MANAGEMENT PHILOSOPHY

Management philosophy refers to the explicit or implicit beliefs of key managers about the nature of the business, its role in society, and the very way that it is run.[2] Management philosophy as it relates to personnel specifically determines the extent to which employees are treated and utilized.

MASLOW'S HIERARCHY OF NEEDS

To establish a sound and effective philosophy, the needs of those that will be affected should be understood first. To better understand this concept, an athletic trainer needs to look no further than the original hierarchy of needs that was created by Maslow to identify those components that are essential for human motivational needs (Figure 11-1).[3] In this pyramidal hierarchical approach, Maslow identified needs as being physiological, safety, belonging, self-esteem, and self-actualizing.

Physiological needs refer to the most basic requirements of survival: food, shelter, and warmth. These are provided to employees through earned wages, but will affect each differently depending on individual requirements. *Safety needs* relate to those concerns that an employee may have about personal safety against theft, physical or emotional abuse, or fears that one must overcome regarding job stability and growth. As a manager, a person can play a role in ensuring certain levels of safety by always taking employees' fears and concerns for these needs very seriously.

Often the feeling that a person has of *belonging* to a group or organization can determine the level of performance put forth. This need of belonging is seen as Maslow's central level of motivation. As a manager, a person can help to establish these emotions through the implementation of both formal and informal group activities and projects.[4]

Self-esteem and *self-actualization* are needs that people possess typically following the successful attainment of the basic requirements of safety and belonging. Self-esteem needs of an employee can be met by providing the employee with additional opportunities to contribute on a more individualized basis. Sending an athletic trainer to a continuing education course and then having him or her come back to the clinic to share that information or new technique with the rest of the staff is an example of achieving self-esteem needs.

The need to achieve the level of self-actualization is very different than that of self-esteem. Here, an individual's goal is to have an internal feeling of success and accomplishment. Because these individuals wish to continue to contribute to organizations, they truly make attempts to challenge themselves to reach higher levels of performance and completeness.

MANAGEMENT STYLE

As a general rule, managers can be interpreted as demonstrating one of three management styles: autocratic, laissez faire, or democratic. Although no one style can be considered better than another, specific circumstances or situations may call for a specific style in order to achieve optimal results of satisfaction.

An autocratic manager is one who makes decisions with little or no input from others within the organization. We know this as the traditional, dictatorship type approach. Though the autocratic manager ultimately determines judgment on his or her own, it does not rule out the fact that this person has not considered the consequences of the decision nor those who will be affected either directly or indirectly.

By contrast, a democratic approach to management encourages staff input and participation in the decision-making process. Here, collaborative efforts are utilized to determine the best possible approach to a solution. Although staff members enjoy this type of management style, managers should be cautioned that regularly *not* using staff suggestions after requesting input can create adverse reactions among employees. Thus, the democratic leadership style will only appear as a front to an actual autocratic approach.

A laissez faire management style is one that recognizes and is supportive of employee input but one in which the ultimate decision may not necessarily be based upon requested information or suggestions that were gathered. This type of leadership approach is not strictly autocratic or democratic, but instead lies somewhere in the middle. It often results in no decision and issues may be left to die, or possibly multiply into larger problems.

FUNCTIONS OF A MANAGER

Although acting as a manager can appear to be quite different from one organization to another, there are certain entities or functions that a person must perform on a daily basis regardless of where he or she is employed. These functions are planning, organizing, directing, and controlling (Figure 11-2).[5]

Planning

Planning simply refers to the process of deciding "what to do" and "how to do it." This involves not only preparation, but insight into the outcomes of the ultimate decision or product. This function requires those involved to present all of the possible outcomes and prepare for the worse possible case scenarios that could occur. McFarland lists the following questions that a person should ask when in the stages of planning:[1]

1. How long do we have before definite action must take place?
2. Have we tried anything like this before?
3. What makes this situation so urgent?
4. Whom do we have available to help us with this work?
5. What additional resources are available?
6. Have we really succeeded in defining the problem?
7. Where can we get more information?
8. What is our ultimate goal?
9. Who will ultimately be affected by this outcome?

Organizing

The process of organizing is an essential function of a manager. Organizing is the ability to divide up work and allocate it to the appropriate personnel. A manager must realize that support staff is of vital importance and may be of assistance in completing assignments. The process of relaying work to others is referred to as delegation, and will be discussed later in this chapter.

Directing

Directing means ensuring that those who are executing a plan know what to do and in fact are doing it. In order to be a successful director, a person might need to take more of an autocratic approach to management style. Assigning responsibilities and deadlines are examples of directing.

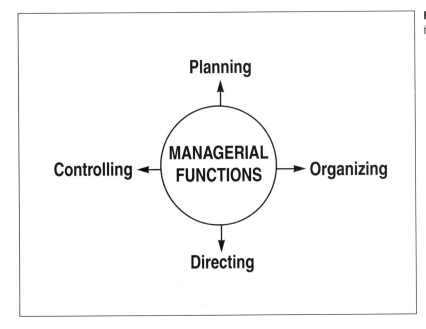

Figure 11-2. Essential functions of a manager.

Controlling

Often, circumstances present that were unplanned or uncontrollable. This can happen regardless of efficient planning, organization, and direction. It is the responsibility of the manager to function in a way to see that any variations in the original plan are kept under control. When unforeseen cases do exist, the main goal is to stay within acceptable limits of change as compared to the initial plan of action.

ROLES AND RESPONSIBILITIES OF A MANAGER

A role is defined as a set of related activities or behaviors associated with a particular position in an organization.[1,5] Although at times a job description will specifically identify the role of a manager, in general there are some common responsibilities that managers in different clinical facilities will share.

Because a personnel manager's role is to manage people, he or she has a responsibility to his or her employees. The necessary skills that a person needs to successfully accomplish employee-related issues will be discussed later in this chapter. If a manager is not also the owner of the facility, then a responsibility will lie in keeping the owner(s) informed of managerial decisions and clinical facility status.

The majority of business derived from a clinical facility occurs as a result of providing a service to a community. Therefore, another responsibility of a manager is to ensure that his or her facility is meeting the needs of the local community. On a larger scale, a facility should also be operating along the lines of agreement with the profession and with society as a whole. This in part serves as a responsibility of a manager who is overseeing a clinical staff.

KEYS TOWARD EFFECTIVE MANAGEMENT OF PERSONNEL

It can be said that successful managers are born, not bred. Yet, it is believed that there are a number of characteristics that can lead to effectiveness in managing people. Competency, motivation, and a desire to succeed appear to be a common ground for successful man-

---

Table 11-1
Key Elements of a Successful Manager

1. Personality
2. Understanding human behavior
3. Communication
4. Influence, leadership, and power
5. Decision-making skills
6. Creativity and innovation
7. Commitment to completion of tasks
8. Conflict management and resolution
9. Stress management
10. Fairness

agers. Although managers may present with different styles and approaches, the following characteristics have been found to be key elements of a successful manager (Table 11-1).

Personality

Empirically, many people believe that an individual's personality has much to do with behavior, performance, and success. Athletic trainers have shown that acceptable and enjoyable personalities have led to increases in rehabilitation compliance with athletes.[6,7] Assuming this to be a contagious characteristic, it would be expected that employee productivity would also be influenced if that person's manager is well-liked.

Understanding Human Behavior

The most important resource for a manager is people. They are the employees who help to control all of the other resources such as money, supplies, and information. The ability to understand human behavior will allow a manager to predict what others will do, and to possibly influence them in decision-making processes. More importantly, a manager should make every effort to provide positive reinforcement when such acknowledgment is warranted.

Communication

Throughout this text the importance of effective communication is emphasized. From a managerial standpoint, effective communication can occur in a verbal or written manner. In today's society, the capability of using advanced technological measures makes it much easier to convey a message to anyone in the world at any time. The key to effective communication, however, is realizing that communication is a two-way road. Therefore, it is imperative that the manager listens to the ideas, thoughts, and feelings of each employee to better understand whether or not the existing levels of communication within a clinical facility are adequate or not. Maintaining an open-door policy remains the best approach to employer receptiveness. Holding regular forums that allow for employees to express their concerns may also be helpful.

Influence, Leadership, and Power

During the course of an average day, a manager may influence or be influenced about a certain administrative decision or action. Influence is referred to as the process of getting others to behave as one would like them to behave. To do so, a person must exert leadership skills. Leadership is a type of influence wherein one individual has influence over a group that motivates them to perform in a certain way. Although this position may be in existence by the very nature of the organizational structure, being unable to exert leadership makes it difficult for that person to influence subordinates. The actual capacity to which a person influences can be seen as a form of power that is exemplified.[5]

Decision-Making Skills

As previously mentioned, managers must make decisions on a regular basis. Not only are there different styles of leadership and communication that lead to the ability to solve problems, but some important skills also serve as the backbone for "deciding how one should decide."

Whereas the process of delegating tasks to others may free up a manager to attend to additional matters, it does not relieve him or her of the responsibilities regarding the assignment. The process of delegating without abdication is a difficult one for many. Few people like to bestow complete authority upon others if they will continue to hold an obligatory role in the final decision. It should be remembered that employees who feel as though they have been given a level of trust see that as a token of opportunity and appreciation. And, in that, will typically behave in such a way that produces optimal levels of effort.

Creativity and Innovation

Stagnancy has never been a quality of successful corporations. Although a person's final product may remain the same, the road taken to get to that point must constantly be re-evaluated and re-assessed. A good manager must always know his or her market and what the competitors are doing. The demand to find managers who strive to be creative and innovative is great. To enhance a person's potential to find new and better ways to perform, managers should continue to look to team members for input.

Commitment to Completion of a Task

Being the nicest person and having the best ideas does not always make for a good manager. One of the critical components to being successful and believable in any profession is the ability to follow through with promises and commitments. When voices of authority talk, people tend to listen. As a manager, the mechanism of setting out to complete a task should be followed through to its entirety. Failure, although not often welcomed, may at least signify a completion of a plan.

Conflict Management and Resolution

In any setting where two or more people may retain different ideas and values, conflicts are sure to occur. You have probably heard the phrase, "it is okay to agreeably disagree." This simply means that everyone does not have the same opinions. If everyone did, the world would not be an exciting place to live. In business, and especially from a managerial point of view, conflicts need to be resolved. Moreover, conflicts should be resolved in a nonthreatening way. It is important to remember that the solution to every conflict is not whether a winner and a loser emerge. Instead, involved parties should focus on ways to stimulate problem-solving efforts so as to better the overall big picture.[8]

The ways of minimizing organizational conflict are as varied as the causes, sources, and contexts. In general, there are three approaches to managing conflict. The first, withdrawal, is more of a strategic technique. Many times one party will withdraw from a discussion for no other reason than to move forward and avoid an issue or unnecessary conflict that is time and energy consuming. This method does not always work, however, if both parties insist on a final result in their favor.[1]

Another way of managing conflict is through a win-lose or power-based strategy. In this case, power, authority, and persuasiveness take a leading role. Employees often resent this

---

Table 11-2
Principal Steps to Follow When Attempting to Reach a Win-Win Result Following a Conflict

1. Clarify the common purpose
2. Keep the discussion relevant
3. Get agreement on terminology
4. Avoid abstract principles; concentrate on the facts
5. Look for potential trade-offs
6. Listen
7. Avoid debating tactics; use persuasive tactics
8. Keep in mind the personal element
9. Use logic logically
10. Seek integrated solutions

---

approach because they may feel as though they have their backs to the wall from the very beginning of the negotiation. This approach can also be excessively timely and costly, and it ultimately leads to the presence of a very unhappy party who has been deemed the loser.[9,10]

Yet a third approach to managing conflict is known as a collaborative or third party intervention method. In this case, the goal is to come to a judgment or decision that is pleasing to both sides. This is sometimes called a compromise. In the most difficult situations, a third party, or mediator/arbitrator, may be asked to hear the arguments of both sides and give a final ruling.[1,9] Levenstein, in the nursing literature, suggests some principles that should be followed in an attempt to reach a win-win outcome (Table 11-2).[11]

Stress Management

Both physical and emotional stress is a part of everyday life. Although no one is immune to "stressors," it becomes incumbent upon everyone to create outlets to control the build-up of these stressors. The American Heart Association found that even monks living in monasteries with higher echelon responsibilities were three times as likely to develop coronary artery disease than those monks in the same monastery, but whom carry less responsibility.[12] As a manager, a person's job regularly involves pressures from within an organization. In fact, many stressful situations center around the pursuit of success. These pressures combined with those of everyday home life, may lead to a decline in a person's mental and physical health status. Health care professionals are very susceptible to stress because of the types of clients they must deal with.

Each person must be responsible for identifying a successful method for preventing the excessive build-up of bodily stressors. For some, this might be listening to music or reading a book. For others, daily exercise or meditation may work. Other techniques include visual imagery, relaxation techniques, controlled breathing techniques, and even a complete change of environment. One must learn to separate a patient's problem from his or her own personal life in order to keep work-related stress in balance.

Fairness

Policy and procedure manuals are designed to set forth rules for everyone to follow.

However, these rules can quickly become overwhelming and over-protective. In such a case, a manager may play the role of interpreter. A manager may also delegate assignments and or employee benefits on various occasions. It becomes extremely important that a manager exhibits equitable behavior and decisions among his or her staff. Perhaps nothing can destroy the cohesiveness of a department more than when staff members feel as though they are being discriminated against or treated unfairly. All efforts should be made by a manager to treat each individual with fairness and avoid favoritism at all costs.

EVALUATION OF EMPLOYEE PERFORMANCE LEVELS

Beer et al state that managers ordinarily list the following attributes and behavior they desire to have among the people they supervise:[2]

- Initiative
- Dependability
- Willingness to take responsibility
- Loyalty to the company and to managers
- Willingness to suggest changes and improvements in the job
- Adaptability and flexibility
- Competence

To adequately assess these and other performance-related activities of an employee, a manager or company should establish a cohesive process to evaluate employees. This may be referred to as an evaluation, an assessment, or even a performance appraisal. Regardless, the intent should be to provide greater objectivity with respect to the judgment of a person's ability to handle a job task. Doing this on a regular basis not only serves as a monitoring process for management, but also as a goal-setting device for an employee.[1] New employees should undergo formal evaluation after the first 6 weeks to 2 months on the job. All employees should undergo formal evaluation on a yearly basis.

Walter advocates that a single performance tool may not adequately measure performance for all employees, thus the design of such a tool should be focused on the standard for performance relative to the job, not the individual.[4] Furthermore, she suggests the following principles to be used as guidelines for the development of a meaningful appraisal system:

1. Develop a valid process—base on job description
2. Develop a reliable process—include self-evaluation
3. Develop an acceptable process—schedule well in advance
4. Develop a fair process—discuss all results
5. Develop a meaningful process—plan for future growth and/or improvement
6. Develop a system that incorporates assessments from all parties served by the employee—may include peer review
7. Build an appraisal system that fits the needs of the department—practical in nature
8. Performance appraisal tools do not assess job performance in its totality—but should suggest indications for promotion
9. Develop a tool that works—have a method to evaluate its effectiveness
10. There are pitfalls in performance assessment—may not positively reward excellence in performance, nor less than average performance

11. Everyone has weaknesses—but do these weaknesses prevent proper completion of job description
12. Be creative—it is usually easier and more effective to retrain than to fire and hire

SUMMARY

Athletic trainers may find themselves in positions of management as their roles in the clinical setting continue to grow. Therefore it is important to have a baseline knowledge of the various styles and philosophy associated with personnel management. Planning, organizing, directing, and controlling are essential functions of a manager. In addition, to be successful, a person needs to possess many different characteristics that would allow for optimal employee/employer relationships.

Study Questions

1. In your own words, how would you define the term "management"?
2. What examples might you think of as a manager of an outpatient clinical setting to enable your staff members to meet their needs according to Maslow's hierarchy?
3. What type of management style do you most often use: autocratic, democratic, or laissez faire? Can you think of any circumstances in which a different style might better suit the situation?
4. List the four essential functions of a manager and explain how each plays an important role with respect to the implementation of a new program.
5. Consider the key elements discussed in this chapter that appear to assist a person in becoming an effective manager of personnel. Design a clinical project in which each of these elements might play a significant role in the ultimate success of the project. Can you think of any other elements that might also be helpful?
6. Assume that you are a manager of a clinical facility and have been given the task of evaluating the performance of all of the staff athletic trainers. Design a plan, including a performance appraisal form, that would help you successfully accomplish this task. What guidelines should you follow during this process?

References

1. McFarland DE. *Management Principles and Practices.* 4th ed. New York, NY: Macmillan Publishing Co, Inc; 1974.
2. Beer M, Spector B, Lawrence PR, Mills DQ, Walton RE. *Human Resource Management.* New Yrok, NY: The Free Press, A Division of Macmillan, Inc; 1985.
3. Maslow A. A theory of human motivation. *Psych Rev.* 1943;50:370-396.
4. Walter J. *Physical Therapy Management: An Integrated Science.* St. Louis, Mo: C.V. Mosby; 1993.

5. Reitz HJ, Jewell LN. *Managing*. Glenview, Ill: Scott, Foresman and Company; 1985.

6. Fisher AC, Hoisington LL. Injured athletes' attitudes and judgments toward rehabilitation adherence. *J Ath Train*. 1993;28:48-54.

7. Fisher AC, Scriber KC, Matheny ML, Alderman MH, Bitting LA. Enhancing athletic injury rehabilitation adherence. *J Ath Train*. 1993;28:312-318.

8. Jandt FE, Gillette P. *Win-Win Negotiating*. New York, NY: 1985:24-37.

9. Nosse LJ, Friberg DG. *Management Principles for Physical Therapists*. Baltimore, Md: Williams & Wilkins; 1992.

10. Schatzki M, Tamborlane TA. Negotiation strategies for conflict resolution. *Caring*. 1988;Feb:71-74.

11. Levenstein A. Negotiation vs. confrontation. *Nursing Management*. 1984;15:52-53.

12. Randall CB. *The Folklore of Management*. Boston, Mass: Little, Brown and Company; 1961.

Suggested Readings

Bohannon RW. The performance appraisal: considerations for supervisors and staff. *Clin Management*. 1987;7:10-13.

Davis GL, Bordieri JE. Perceived autonomy and job satisfaction in occupational therapists. *Am J Occup Ther*. 1988;42:591-595.

Drucker PF. *The Practice of Management*. New York, NY: Harper and Row Publishers; 1986.

Emery M, Walter J. Self-assessment: performance appraisal system in a time of increasing specialization. *Phys Ther*. 1981;61:702.

Gordon IM. Our policies are tough, but our staff is happy. *Medical Economics*. 1988;Aug:85-89.

Lachman VD. Increasing productivity through performance evaluation. *J Nursing Admin*. 1984;14:7-14.

McCord R. Perfect employees are not born, you train them. *Physician's Management*. 1988;Nov:53-57.

McNeil LL, Gutterud SR. Employee satisfaction: the bottom line. *PT Today*. 1991;Spring:21-26.

Metzger SG. Super staffing: a competitive edge. *PT Forum*. 1992;Apr:24-25,36.

Roseman E. Collaborative negotiation: getting agreements that last. *Med Lab Observer*. 1986;Feb:71-74.

Schermerhorn JR. Improving health care productivity through high-performance managerial development. *Health Care Manage Rev*. 1987;12:49-55.

Schutle JE. Let patients tell you how to make your practice better. *Medical Economics*. 1988;Sept:179-186.

CHAPTER

12

Communication Skills in Clinical Athletic Training

Jeff G. Konin, MEd, ATC, MPT

OBJECTIVES

Upon completion of this chapter, the student will be able to accomplish the following:

1. Distinguish between verbal and nonverbal communication

2. Demonstrate the various types of nonverbal communication

3. Identify keys to successful communication

4. Recognize the role of listening in effective communication

C ommunication plays a major role in determining the success of any task that is carried out, regardless of profession. Of all the skills necessary to become an effective health care provider, the ability to effectively communicate may just be the most important. The act of both sending and receiving messages in a manner that facilitates comprehension and subsequent positive actions can be the difference between successful and unsuccessful rehabilitation, agreements and disagreements, or positive and negative predicaments.

Historically, athletic trainers have been effective communicators in the traditional settings. For the most part, these skills have been inherently developed to assist an athlete in his or her attempt to achieve optimal levels of performance.[1-5]

When dealing with clients, the clinical, industrial, and corporate settings pose a new and different challenge for the athletic trainer. Ranges in the levels of motivation may be greater than when working solely with the highly competitive athletic population. In addition, cultural diversity, chronological and physiological age representation, and the health status of individuals being cared for in the nontraditional settings require the athletic trainer to accommodate to various lifestyles and personalities.

While knowledge and experience are always important components of delivering quality care, the ability to transfer this knowledge in a manner in which a client can comfortably understand the essential elements associated with successful rehabilitation is the hallmark of a good clinician. It has been said that "people don't care how much you know, until they know how much you care." This thought holds especially true in health care. A clinician must gain confidence and trust from a client before adequate compliance to a regimen can be expected. This can be accomplished through effective communication.

The goal of this chapter is to familiarize the reader with the different methods of communication that can be utilized to enhance professional interaction. These skills can be utilized to enhance clinician–client interactions, professional relationships, and even personal communication.

TYPES OF COMMUNICATION

Verbal

When one person speaks to another, verbal communication is taking place. However, the mere fact that a voice is projecting a sound does not constitute the effective delivery of a message from one party to another. For example, if someone spoke to you in a language that was foreign to your vocabulary, you would not be able to comprehend the message regardless of how slowly or clearly the person spoke. When a language is spoken that is familiar, it can only be effective in its delivery if it contains what are known as the five Cs of communication:[6]

1. Complete
2. Clear
3. Concise
4. Courteous
5. Cohesive

The following example shows how the five Cs play a role in clinical athletic training: An athletic trainer is designing a home program for a client with a quadricep strain. First, the exercises that will be implemented must be explained in detail so that the client is fully aware of the movements for each. In order for the client to be able to perform these exercises correctly, the explanation of each must be clear and concise. The clinician must then be courteous, possibly allowing time for questions that the client may have with respect to the individual exercises. Not allowing time for questions may result in miscommunication. Lastly, it is important for the clinician to explain the exercises in a logical and meaningful manner. For example, it would make more sense to first demonstrate and explain to the client how to perform a "quadricep set" isometric contraction, and then progress to a straight leg raise while building on the initial exercise. It also helps to address all important details at the appropriate time intervals. If the athletic trainer wanted the client to have the contralateral knee bent at 90 degrees of flexion during the straight leg raise exercise, it would be much better to demonstrate and explain this at the time of the exercise as opposed to when the client is leaving the facility and the ATC finds him- or herself saying, "Oh, by the way, bend your opposite knee when you perform the straight leg raise."

In health care, verbal communication may occur: 1) to establish clinician–client rapport, 2) to obtain information concerning client status, 3) to relay pertinent information to another health professional, and 4) to give instructions to the client or caregivers.[7] Regardless of the circumstance, attention to detail must be followed. In fact, Sanson-Fisher and Maguire have stated that one of the primary reasons that clients may not follow instructions given to them by a health professional is due to a lack of effectiveness in verbal communication.[8]

Purtilo further believes that the success of verbal communication depends on several important factors that include the way in which the material is actually presented, the attitude of the presenter, the tone and volume of the voice, and the degree to which the presenter and the receiver are able to listen effectively.[7]

The difference between the mechanism by which one verbally communicates information to a peer versus how one delivers the same message to a patient with no medical background must be understood. When explaining to an athletic training student how ultrasound works for the treatment of adhesive capsulitis, an athletic trainer might say, "electrical energy is converted into acoustical energy by means of a reverse piezoelectric effect...thus resulting in a thermal response which increases collagen elasticity." When asked by a client how ultrasound works, the same athletic trainer might respond by simply stating, "sound waves are used to heat up the tissue which will help us to stretch it." Both responses are correct, but have been tailored to the appropriate level of listening and understanding. An assessment of the level of the listener is always important so that the athletic trainer does not unintentionally insult a person as a result of trying to simplify an explanation. For example, if the same client in this case was, in fact, an electrical engineer, he or she might be more interested in knowing what level of intensity the ATC is using while delivering the modality.

Nonverbal

One does not always have to speak in a verbal manner to convey a message. Perceptions, images, and opinions can be formulated merely by watching the actions of a person. As will be discussed in Chapter 13, the physical appearance and dress of an athletic trainer can portray an image and a message to clients and co-workers. There are many other means by which one can communicate through nonverbal mechanisms. It is imperative for the athletic trainer to become familiar with these nonverbal means of communication in order to facilitate positive responses through appropriate measures. Displaying nonverbal communication, even unintentionally, can subtly create a communication barrier that is non-conducive to the environment.

Body Language

Most nonverbal communication takes place in the form of body language. This is a general term that describes how an individual uses his or her body to demonstrate feelings and expressions. People have used body language since infancy, e.g., by smiling or frowning to communicate to parents. Essentially, most nonverbal communications through body language are unconscious, learned movements. For example, an athletic trainer may yawn while his or her client is explaining how he was initially injured. Even though the ATC may be listening very intently, the client will perceive the yawn to mean that he or she is tired and not interested in the medical history. This is another example of how a facial expression can be used to communicate a message. Therefore, learning to control body language can be a tremendous advantage to a clinician.

Eye Contact

Eye contact is also considered to reflect a message on behalf of the clinician. If, for example, a clinician does not establish good eye contact with a client during treatment, the client may interpret simultaneous verbal instructions as not being important. Direct eye contact tends to send a message that equates to a higher level of importance. However, while establishing eye contact is good, one should take care not to create a long, uncomfortable stare. This tends to intimidate some, while others may actually see it as an invasion of privacy.[7,9]

Use of Touch

The use of touch is also a strong form of nonverbal communication. Athletic trainers' jobs involve a lot of hands-on type activity. Physical contact in the form of touch is perceived by clients in many ways. When dealing with clients in the health environment, physical touch often equates to trust, caring, reassurance, understanding, and interest. The initiation of a gentle, yet firm touch can also help to establish a rapport with clientele.[9] Nonetheless, the clinician should be careful to avoid overpowering another individual through this mechanism of communication. There are some people who may, in fact, become more uncomfortable with a clinican's touch. These people may not be reassured, and instead they too may feel an invasion of privacy. Whether or not to use touch as a means of nonverbal communication is a difficult decision that the athletic trainer must learn to make when dealing with assorted personalities.

Positioning

How a person positions him- or herself when communicating with others may also influence the comfort perception of the receiver. Natural, face-to-face conversation usually occurs with 2 to 5 feet between the individuals. Typically, as an individual moves more to the side of another person, the receiver gets more comfortable with a closer distance of communication. Territorial boundaries should be established to ensure a comfortable environment as well as to facilitate optimal performance.

Maintaining a position during communication also establishes a sense of consistency. This is opposed to movements either toward or away from a client. Moving closer to a person may signal a feeling of acceptance and trust. By contrast, movement away from a person often denotes disinterest and impatience, which can quickly destroy any previous successful attempts at communication.

In addition, a clinician who positions him- or herself above a client in such a way that he or she is looking down at the person exemplifies a position of superiority. This can make the person who is looking up feel very insecure and uncomfortable, not the scenario that anyone would like to create. Many physicians have said that they will sit on stools and place patients on examining tables when dialogue occurs so that the patients do not feel intimidated during office visits.

In addition to general positioning of oneself, a person's specific posture also sends a message; for example, how a clinician uses his or her evaluation skills when differentially diagnosing an injury. Observation of posture and alignment of a joint or structure can play a key role in a final assessment. Athletic trainers have been taught to recognize certain postures or "carrying positions" of individuals and how these changes relate to injury. For example, an athletic trainer may observe a client walk through the facility while touch down weight bearing and avoiding heel strike. This indicates to the ATC that the ground reaction forces associated with weight bearing on the heel may be painful to this individual. The clinician can observe a person's postural change and interpret the meaning of the deviation. However, clients can assess postural changes in the clinician as well. These bodily alterations many times are performed and presented unknowingly. Therefore, while a clinician, or client, may be thinking one thing, and possibly even speaking to the same tune, his or her posture may say something entirely different.

Gestures

Possibly the most obvious and commonly used method of communicating nonverbally is through the use of gestures. Many people use their hands to assist with verbal communication. Often hand movement may be used to emphasize certain points simultaneously with verbal delivery. Gestures have a powerful way of sending a message. For example, think back to when you were a kid. Do you ever remember your dad or mom standing with his or her arms crossed sternly looking at you without saying a word? You knew exactly what kind of thoughts were running through their heads.

Gestures can be used both consciously and unconsciously. When a person is asked a question to which she cannot remember the answer, she may place a finger to her chin and look upwards toward the sky. When someone is nervous, he may involuntarily tap his fingers or jingle change in his pocket. Typically, when people are tense or angry, they will clench their fists and flair their nostrils. These are just some examples of how simple gestures can convey a message.

It is important, however, to assess one's gesture in context with all other verbal and nonverbal expressions prior to making a conclusion as to the meaning of an individual gesture.[9] For instance, a common gesture involves the individual standing with both arms crossed in front of the chest. Depending on the circumstance, this can have one of two meanings. One could be relaxed, smiling and partaking in friendly conversation; another could be angry, taking repeated deep breaths and waiting to speak aggressively. Assessing the environment and the additional portrayals of this person would help to conclude the true meaning of the crossed arms gesture.

Written Communication

Written communication is another form of nonverbal communication. Written communication for the purpose of documentation is discussed in detail in Chapter 15. When working in a clinical setting where an athletic trainer may only see a client a couple times per week, issuing the client a home exercise program in writing serves as a beneficial tool. A form of this nature could be specific to the exercises that were given to a client, and may even include pictorial demonstrations of these exercises.

Many companies have developed computer software exercise programs to assist with client compliance. Others have developed index cards that depict individual exercises. These programs are advantageous to clinicians because they are professionally designed. They are also of help to the client performing the home exercise program. However, the client may need to be supplemented with additional information if a clinician wishes to implement an exercise that is not included in the pre-designed set or software.

When an athletic trainer designs his or her own exercise sheets, it is important for him or her to be clear and concise. Pictures of individual exercises should be accompanied by descriptive explanations. It may be a good idea to have non-health care professionals proofread these forms to see if they can clearly understand how to perform each exercise. It is also important for athletic trainers to remember the specific population they are serving. For instance, if a clinician is working with a geriatric, physically active population, he or she may want to consider using larger font sizes when typesetting. Thus another disadvantage of pre-designed exercise forms are that while they may sufficiently meet the needs of most of the clientele, there will probably be a portion for whom the forms are not appropriate.

Active Listening

Effective communication is only achieved when one party successfully delivers a message and another party successfully receives that very same message. In order to successfully receive a message, the receiver must learn to be an active listener. Too often people listen to others speak, but really do not hear what is being said. Often a listener's attention is not focused on the task of actually listening and processing the message so that it has a meaning.

As a health care provider, it is safe to say that athletic trainers spend a good portion of each day listening to athletes, coaches, and others discussing a wide variety of topics. Even the most effectively delivered message may not be completely communicated to the receiver if the receiver does not actively listen.

What is the difference between simply listening and actively listening? Table 12-1 provides an example of different levels of listening demonstrated by Smith.[10] Of the different levels, Smith believes that health care providers are more involved with analytical, directed, and attentive levels of listening when dealing with patients.

Active listening involves total effort and attention given to a message. It also requires the listener to approach the message with an open mind, as opposed to a preconceived interest or belief with respect to either the delivery or receipt of the message. For a health care provider, it is difficult to ensure that a client actively listens to his or her directions. One method of enhancing the ability of a client to actively listen is to ask him or her to repeat or demonstrate the activity that was just described. If done correctly, the health

Table 12-1
Levels of Listening[10]

1. Analytical—listening for specific kinds of information
2. Directed—listening to answer specific questions
3. Attentive—listening for general information to obtain an overview
4. Exploratory—listening is due to one's own interest
5. Appreciative—listening for pleasure
6. Courteous—listening as a result of feeling obligated
7. Passive—not listening in an attentive manner

care provider can at least be assured of short-term retention of the message. If not done correctly, both parties will become aware of the miscommunication, and usually they will try harder on the next attempt to achieve improved levels of success.

The athletic trainer as a health provider can practice active listening through simple techniques such as repeating a client's statement or question in part or whole when responding with his or her own answer. If, for example, a client asked, "How long will this knee pain last?", the athletic trainer might respond by saying, "How long will your knee pain last? Probably about 2 weeks."

Purtilo lists the following simple steps to improve effective listening:[7]

1. Be selective to what you listen.
2. Concentrate on central themes rather than isolated statements.
3. Judge content rather than style or delivery.
4. Listen with an open mind.
5. Summarize in your own mind what you hear before speaking again.
6. Clarify before proceeding. Do not let vague or incomplete ideas go unattended.

KEYS TO SUCCESSFUL COMMUNICATION

The key to communicating in an effective and successful manner involves the complete interaction between the delivering and receiving of a message. The delivery of a message may be enhanced through the use of both verbal and nonverbal communication methods, so long as the messages being sent through different techniques are actually saying the same thing.

The listener must be active and open minded when receiving a message. Listening always has been and always will be a large component that assists the athletic trainer with his or her daily responsibilities. More and more these days, as a result of health care concerns of the consumer, the athletic trainer needs to spend more time actively listening to his or her clients.

A general rule of thumb to follow when establishing effective communication lines between a client or a co-worker is to recognize that a technique that works with one person may not work with another. This is no different than the rehabilitation protocols that are designed for clients and athletes. Most likely, in one way or another, a protocol for each individual case will need to be modified. Learning to communicate effectively is both an art and a science, and it requires practice and experience in dealing with multiple personalities. Not every person is an ideal candidate for successful communication.

By the very nature of the situation, each client who enters a clinical facility has entered out of necessity as opposed solely to choice. To attend rehabilitation sessions, most times these individuals undergo changes and possibly inconveniences to adjust their schedules accordingly. In addition, many people are experiencing increased levels of pain and discomfort that may be limiting their daily activities. It is important to recognize that these individuals may not present themselves in a "happy-go-lucky" type of mood. By contrast, they may appear angry, frustrated, and even unwilling to communicate.

This presents a challenge for the clinical athletic trainer. Nonetheless, the ability to communicate effectively with the most reluctant person is a characteristic that separates successful professionals from mediocre employees. This is a situation that is often seen in clinical settings and, in fact, is approached differently by the novice and experienced clinician. The novice clinician, who has limited exposure to dealing with uncooperative clients, may choose to reduce his or her effort of communicating, thus giving the client no more help than he or she has attempted to give the clinician. Looking at the overall picture, both parties have set the stage for failure of communication. The negative relationship may lead to a slower rate of recovery and return to daily activities. Rotella has outlined "problem patients" under categories such as "dependent attention-loving patients," "resistant athletes," "childlike patients," "angry patients," and "unmotivated athletes," and offers practical ideas to improve communication with these individuals.[11]

Given the same situation, the experienced clinician realizes that the client may not normally act in this manner. In fact, the verbal and nonverbal expressions of the client are simply a result of the temporary inconvenience. In reality, the client wants to return to normal activity as soon as possible, but has not been faced with this type of situation before and therefore does not know how to react to the circumstances. By continuing open communication and facilitating a positive environment, the experienced clinician is more likely to ameliorate an active approach to rehabilitation for the client.

SUMMARY

Some of the best athletic trainers are not necessarily the most knowledgeable or experienced, but instead the most effective communicators. For athletic trainers to continue to be effective communicators, an understanding of general communication skills must be perceived as a vital component to clinical practice. Recognizing the countless number of individuals whom athletic trainers come in contact with on a daily basis helps the athletic trainer to prepare to use different communication styles and techniques such as verbal and nonverbal methods. The ability to communicate is a learned skill that should not be taken for granted, but instead practiced on an ongoing basis to ensure success.

Study Questions

1. Explain the difference between verbal and nonverbal communication techniques.
2. What are some of the types of nonverbal communication? What are some common types of nonverbal communication that an athletic trainer may

portray that can be perceived either as being negative or uninterested?

3. As an athletic trainer, act out a scene with a partner who plays the role of a client in a clinical setting with acute low back pain. Walk through the process of obtaining a history from the client. Following this scene, have observers discuss your ability to communicate effectively with the client.

4. How would you go about utilizing written communication for your clients in an industrial setting for the assistance of preventive exercise programs? Are there any specific concerns that you may have with respect to the creation of these documents?

5. What is active listening? How is active listening important in achieving successful communication between you and your clients, as well as you and your co-workers?

6. What do you believe are the keys to effective communication? Do you currently practice these components?

7. What components of effective communication do you feel are your strengths? What components do you feel are your weaknesses? How could you implement a strategy to improve upon your communication skills that you have identified as being weaknesses?

8. Upon first meeting a client who has been sent to your facility for the treatment of elbow pain, the client states that he doesn't believe that you can help him, but the doctor wanted him to try rehabilitation. Knowing that you are now working with an individual who has created a communication barrier, how would you approach the situation in order to maximize treatment results?

References

1. DePalma MT, DePalma B. The use of instruction and the behavioral approach to facilitate injury rehabilitation. *J Ath Train*. 1989;24:217-219.

2. Fisher AC. Adherence to sports injury rehabilitation programs. *Sports Med*. 1990:9;151-158.

3. Fisher AC, Hoisington LL. Injured athletes' attitudes and judgments toward rehabilitation adherence. *J Ath Train*. 1993;28:48-54.

4. Fisher AC, Mullins SA, Frye PA. Athletic trainers' attitudes and judgments of injured athletes' rehabilitation adherence. *J Ath Train*. 1993;28:43-47.

5. Fisher AC, Scriber KC, Matheny ML, Alderman MH, Bitting LA. Enhancing athletic injury rehabilitation adherence. *J Ath Train*. 1993;28:312-318.

6. Wilkes M, Crosswait BC. *Professional Development: The Dynamics of Success*. New York, NY:Harcourt Brace Jovanovich; 1991.

7. Purtilo R. *Health Professional and Patient Interaction*. 4th ed. Philadelphia, Pa:WB Saunders Company; 1990.

8. Sanson-Fisher R, Maguire P. Should skills in communicating with patients be taught? *Lancet*. 1980;1:523-526.

9. Scully RM, Barnes ML. *Physical Therapy*. Philadelphia, Pa:JB Lippincott; 1989.

10. Smith E. Improving listening effectiveness. *Tex Med*. 1975;71:98-100.

11. Rotella RJ. Psychological Care of the Injured Athlete. In: Kuland DN, ed. *The Injured Athlete*. 2nd ed. Philadelphia, Pa: JB Lippincott; 1988.

Suggested Readings

Athletic Training and Sports Medicine. Park Ridge, Ill:American Academy of Orthopaedic Surgeons; 1991.

Brinkman R, Kirschner R. *Dealing With People You Can't Stand*. New York, NY: McGraw-Hill; 1994.

Corman LC. The patient knows best. *JAMA*. 1987;257:1225.

Druckman D, Rozelle R, Baxter J. *Nonverbal Communication: Survey, Theory and Research*. Beverly Hills, Calif: Sage Publications; 1982.

King M, Novik L, Citrenbaum C. *Irresistible Communications: Creative Skills for the Health Professional*. Philadelphia, Pa: WB Saunders Co; 1982.

Weiss MR, Troxel RR. Psychology of the injured athlete. *J Ath Train*. 1986;21:104-109.

Clinical Professionalism

Jerome A. "Jai" Isear, MS, PT, ATC

OBJECTIVES

Upon completion of this chapter, the student will be able to accomplish the following:

1. Identify the main components of professionalism

2. Appreciate the differences between the traditional and nontraditional athletic training settings related to the main components of professionalism

3. Explain the important components of the clinician–patient relationship

4. List ways to improve collegial interaction

5. Explain ways to improve commitment to professional growth

6. Describe the suggested attire for the clinical athletic trainer

7. Recognize the importance of punctuality

8. Appreciate the level of responsibility associated with making and maintaining commitments

9. Understand the professional role and limitations of the clinical athletic trainer

The steady influx of athletic training professionals into the nontraditional settings has led athletic trainers to become familiar with new roles and responsibilities. Professionalism is a hallmark that every community or group wishes to achieve to its fullest respect. As athletic trainers journey into new environments such as sports medicine clinics, hospitals, and industrial settings, the area of clinical professionalism presents the athletic trainer with an opportunity to portray his or her profession with a positive image.

More so, it is important to recall that each certified athletic trainer not only represents him- or herself but also represents the profession. On a smaller, yet more personal level, an athletic trainer carries the reputation of his or her graduating institution as well as any mentor who has provided that individual with a recommendation.

As such, this chapter will provide a brief definitional overview of professionalism as well as highlight some of the major components of professionalism as they relate to the clinical athletic trainer. These components include behavior and attitude, attire, hygiene, punctuality, commitment, and an understanding of the athletic trainer's role and related limitations in the clinical setting.

PROFESSIONALISM—CAN IT BE DEFINED?

What is professionalism? How is it defined? Or better yet, can or should it be defined? Reynolds[1] very eloquently suggests that medical professionalism is based on the following set of professional behaviors: "...a nonjudgmental and respectful approach to patients, the pursuit of specialized knowledge and skills with a commitment to excellence and life-long competency, and a collegial and cooperative approach to working with members of a health care team in the delivery of patient care."

Bryan[2] echoes these points with a discussion of the key elements of professionalism as put forth by the American Board of Internal Medicine, including the following: altruism, accountability, excellence, duty, honor, integrity, and respect. One final element of professionalism is peer review. In essence, peer review will serve as a check and balance system to monitor all components of professionalism, and, as Blumenthal[3] suggests, "...to protect consumers against failures of professionalism."

Because of the complexity and potential semantical quandaries associated with the term "professionalism," one should exercise caution when attempting to define the term. Perhaps avoiding an all-inclusive definition and instead emphasizing fundamental components would serve as a more appropriate response. It would behoove one to focus on such words as "excellence," "nonjudgmental," "respect," "altruism," "commitment," and "accountability" because essentially, these are words by which all clinicians should base their clinical practice. A clear understanding of the main components of clinical professionalism is essential before entering the clinical setting.

Professional Behavior and Attitude

Quite commonly, a clinician bases his or her potential for success on his or her own knowledge base or lack thereof. Obviously, a solid knowledge base is required in any health care profession. Of equal, or perhaps even greater importance, however, is an individual's own ability to interact and communicate with both patients and colleagues. This ability is based largely on a person's behavior and attitude in the clinic.

CLINICIAN–PATIENT RELATIONSHIP

When interacting with a patient, generally the ultimate treatment goal of any clinician is to return the patient to his or her premorbid level of function. With the changes occurring within the health care system, however, frequency and duration of treatments have been drastically reduced. As a result, patients are spending less time in the clinic and more time at home with home exercise programs. These programs should ultimately emphasize the importance of patient education. Therefore, perhaps a more important goal upon which to focus for both the novice and experienced clinician would be to endeavor to engage the patient in the rehabilitation process. For without the patient's assistance, his or her rehabilitation potential will most likely be poor.

In order to effectively interact with patients and successfully engage them in the rehabilitation process, a clinician must establish good lines of communication, a hallmark quality of the athletic trainer. The nontraditional setting, however, may pose more of a challenge for the athletic trainer than would the traditional setting, as he or she may not always be dealing with a motivated, athletic population. The typical outpatient population may vary greatly in age, socioeconomic status, desire, and/or incentive to improve, thus placing a great deal of strain on the lines of communication. If the clinician cannot overcome these obstacles and be an effective communicator, he or she will do the patient a disservice. Therefore, in order to facilitate the communication process, the athletic trainer must demonstrate basic behavioral and attitudinal skills, traits, and characteristics, in addition to those discussed by Reynolds and Bryan. A demonstration of self-confidence and a sense of humor are examples of the types of behavior that may need to be exemplified.

Confidence

Confidence, not cockiness, can be a powerful tool for any health care professional. It can help ease patient anxiety as patients tend to be a bit intimidated and scared, especially during the first few treatment sessions. As for the clinician, quite often an outward display of confidence can overshadow inward feelings of incompetence. Feelings of uncertainty or incompetence are not unusual to experience, particularly if the person is a novice clinician. This does not mean, however, that an athletic trainer should fall prey to the "know-it-all syndrome." If an answer is unknown, let that be known. By no means should admitting "I don't know" to a patient's question be interpreted as having a limited knowledge base or a lack of confidence. In fact, the process of obtaining the answer will more often than not turn the situation into a positive learning experience for all people involved. Along these same lines, always explain treatment techniques before implementing them so as to reduce potential patient anxiety. When doing so, as a general rule, present technique explanations in laymen's terms, at least initially. As patient rapport and interest increase or if the patient requests, then offer more technical explanations. This practice, although appearing simplistic at first glance, can truly be challenging as our medical rhetoric is frequently more fluent than that of our English language.

Specifically, confidence can be characterized by a firm handshake upon introduction and by consistent eye contact throughout the treatment session. Confidence is also characterized by assertiveness. Never has this been, or will this be, more important than during the current and future changes in the health care system. From Day 1 to discharge, the rehabilitation team must establish, maintain, and frequently reinforce the importance of patient compliance. This can be accomplished by simply asking the patient to explain and demonstrate the components of his or her home exercise program at the outset of each treatment session. Blatant flaws in and inconsistencies with explanations and demonstrations will send a quick message to the patient that noncompliance will not be tolerated. Please note that in no way should assertiveness and confidence replace empathy, altruism, and respect for the patient. Conversely, let it be known that the days of leading a patient by the hand through the rose garden are numbered.

Sense of Humor

In the clinical setting, the athletic trainer may not always be dealing with a motivated, athletic population. Because of this difference in patient population, the atmosphere in the clinical, nontraditional setting tends to be a bit more formal than in the traditional training room environment, and the athletic trainer's conduct should therefore reflect this level of formality. Nevertheless, displaying a good sense of humor in the clinical setting is a necessity for the athletic trainer. Humor helps to decrease tension between the patient and the clinician, thus providing for a looser, more relaxed atmosphere. It is a known fact that rehabilitation alone can be quite boring at times. The clinician, therefore, can and should serve as a catalyst for making it fun. The rehabilitation process must be a positive experience for the patient. Otherwise, he or she will lose interest. Losing interest in therapy can equate to decreased compliance and ultimately decreased rehabilitation potential.

Humor can also assist a clinician in coping with and preventing burnout. As discussed in Chapter 5, occupational burnout is not uncommon to the athletic trainer. It should be stressed, however, that an athletic trainer who chooses to use humor as an avenue for environmental relaxation should emphasize wit and deemphasize potentially offensive joke telling. Jokes and insults related to gender, race, religion, and culture have no place in any professional athletic training setting.

COLLEGIAL RELATIONSHIPS

Another important aspect of professional behavior and attitude is the development and maintenance of strong working relationships between athletic trainers and other health care professionals. This requires the athletic trainer to possess a positive attitude, an open mind, and a commitment to professional growth.

Positive Attitude

A positive attitude is essential for success in any and every aspect of life. Unfortunately, negative criticism comes much easier than does positive criticism. In addition, negative comments appear to be contagious. Quite frankly, it is difficult to respect a colleague whose pessimism consistently overshadows his or her optimism. Furthermore, if an athletic trainer is unhappy and pessimistic, it will most likely show during interactions with patients as well as with other health care professionals. Remember, complaining fosters negativity, and negativity, in turn, impedes productivity.

Open-Minded

Another important factor that facilitates successful collegial relationships is open-mindedness. As such, the athletic trainer should never enter a clinic "wearing blinders." Much like negativity, close-mindedness is a self-limiting factor. Therefore, the athletic trainer should endeavor to be positively critical instead of negatively critical. Colleagues should possess a willingness to challenge and to be challenged that will ultimately stimulate intellectual growth and promote respect. All clinicians have strengths and weaknesses. If the strengths are shared among colleagues, the weaknesses will undoubtedly diminish.

Commitment to Professional Growth

One final aspect of professional behavior and attitude as it relates to collegial interaction is a commitment to professional growth. This commitment can and should be made in several different areas, the first of which involves professional memberships. Membership with the athletic training associations at the state, district, and national levels, as well as with the American College of Sports Medicine, allows the athletic trainer to be informed about, and contribute to, the current and future status of the profession. Moreover, it encourages the development of comradery within the profession, a unique characteristic of the NATA.

Another area where commitments should be made is in continuing education. Continuing education is a means in which clinicians can strengthen potential weaknesses, provide further intellectual stimulation among colleagues, and potentially enhance the quality of patient care. It challenges the athletic trainer to question why he or she performs certain treatment techniques and not others. It also allows the clinician to break out of and/or improve upon treatment and administrative ruts, habits, and protocols.

A final commitment should be made to the research process. This can be a rewarding experience not only for the researchers but also for the entire profession. Instead of relying on the "regulars" to answer questions, athletic trainers should strive to answer questions themselves. Athletic trainers need to engage themselves in the research process in order to help the profession, and in doing so it will enable them to support or refute clinical observations, biases, and self-proclaimed theories. Athletic trainers should endeavor to be leaders, not followers.

ATTIRE AND HYGIENE

Traditionally, the prototype athletic trainer has been pictured as wearing a T-shirt, shorts, and tennis shoes, which in many cases is appropriate for outdoor athletic event coverage. Unfortunately, use of this attire has carried over to the continuing education courses as well as to state, district, and national conventions. However, with the increasing publicity and recognition of athletic trainers, the importance of a more professional appearance has increased. As the athletic trainer continues to expand into different settings, increased emphasis must be placed on his or her appearance in order to develop and maintain a sense of pride, identity, and respect of the profession among the general public, colleagues, and other health care professionals.

As previously discussed, the clinical setting is often more formal than the traditional setting, and the athletic trainer's appearance must reflect a certain level of formality. As

Figure 13-1. Example of professional attire for male athletic trainers in the clinical setting.

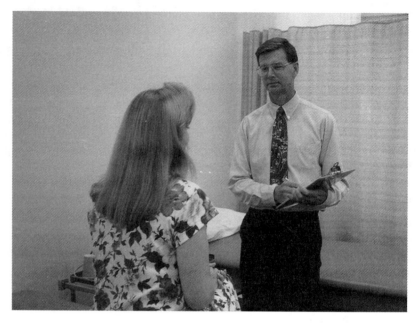

such, the athletic trainer should be easily distinguishable from patients and should reflect a similar appearance to other members of the rehabilitation team, including physical therapists, physical therapist assistants, exercise physiologists, and aides. This requires adherence to specific attire and hygiene.

Attire

Many facilities have dress code policies with which a clinician must comply. A few guidelines should be followed, however, in the event that the dress code is left to the discretion of the clinician. The goal for the athletic trainer should be to portray a clean-cut clinical professional. As a general rule, the "casual look" is discouraged, such as jeans, shorts, and T-shirts. Tennis shoes are discouraged unless approved by an individual facility, or in the case that the clinician has associated low back or lower extremity pathology.

Suggestions for the male include a dress or casual dress shirt with a collar (a tie is recommended), dress or casual dress slacks with a belt, socks, and dress or casual dress shoes, either of the loafer or lace-up type. Open-toed or open-backed shoes are unacceptable. Dress boots are acceptable if in good taste and style (Figure 13-1).

Suggestions for the female include a blouse, shirt, or sweater with dress or casual dress slacks, socks or hose, and low-heeled dress or casual dress shoes. Open-toed or open-backed shoes are unacceptable. Dresses and skirts are acceptable if of the appropriate length (knee length or lower), however denim skirts or revealing slit dresses and skirts are unacceptable.

All clothing should adequately cover the body so as to minimize the display of undergarments and anterior thorax. Likewise, clothing should fit properly and should be neither excessively tight nor excessively loose and baggy. Clothes should not display any slogans or printed materials unless specifically related to the facility or profession. Also, proper undergarments should be worn at all times, and jewelry should not be excessive or gaudy. When appropriate, name tags should be worn to further distinguish clinicians from patients and other personnel. Most importantly, the clinician should look and feel comfortable so that his or her attire does not interfere with patient care. Care should be taken, however, so that professional appearance has not been sacrificed for comfort levels.

Hygiene

Personal hygiene for the athletic trainer and any health care professional should resemble that which is characteristic of any responsible adult. Hair should be neatly groomed, and, if shoulder length or longer, hair should be neatly styled and pulled back from the face. Styling gels and sprays should be kept to a minimum. Beards, mustaches, and sideburns should be of the appropriate length and neatly groomed. Fingernails should be kept clean and of an appropriate length in order to avoid potential injury to patients. In addition, the clinician should avoid excessive use of cosmetics, perfumes, and colognes. Also, in order to portray a healthy image, the athletic trainer should regularly engage in proper dietary and fitness habits.

While in the clinic, because of frequent contact with a variety of patients, all health care professionals should engage in frequent hand washing so as to minimize and/or prevent contraction and proliferation of any communicable diseases. Strict adherence to the Occupational Safety and Health Administration (OSHA) regulations is essential.

Punctuality

Another important component of professionalism is punctuality. As is the case with wearing proper attire and practicing proper hygiene, being punctual should be a characteristic of any responsible adult. Whether related to work shifts, meetings, or deadlines, punctuality is assumed and expected of every health care professional. Of course, unpreventable setbacks may present from time to time. When this occurs, all people who are directly involved should be informed of delays so that alternative plans may be made. This is simply an act of common courtesy. Repeated tardiness, however, is a sign of irresponsibility, and is therefore inexcusable. It reflects a lack of respect for the job, patients, and colleagues, among others. The necessary steps can be taken to prevent tardiness and to ensure punctuality (e.g., utilize business planners, set watches and clocks ahead 5–10 minutes). Punctuality can mean the difference between a noteworthy employee and a mediocre employee.

Commitments

Closely related to punctuality is commitment. It, too, is expected of any responsible adult. Once a commitment is made, it should be maintained until it is completed. If for some uncontrollable reason a commitment must be broken, the clinician should proceed with the understanding of how all parties will be affected. If at all possible, broken commitments should be accompanied by giving adequate notice. Reneging on a commitment reflects poorly on the athletic trainer, both personally and professionally. Most importantly, it signifies a lack of dependability, one of the "3 Ds" (dedication, dependability, and diligence) associated with being a distinguished athletic trainer. Repeated breach of commitment will result in a loss of respect and can quickly create a loss of cohesiveness among colleagues.

Understanding of Role and Related Limitations

From a professional standpoint, the athletic trainer must fully understand his or her role in order to successfully function in the clinical setting. The trainer should keep in mind that he or she is not in the traditional athletic training domain. Moreover, it must be understood that in the clinical setting, the athletic trainer may not "call the shots," depending on individual state law. Ergo, the athletic trainer's frustrations must not be voiced within the clinic during treatment hours as this is neither the time nor the place to discuss such issues. Instead, the athletic trainer should use resources that are designed for discussion of such issues. Examples of appropriate resources might be task forces and committees at the facility, state, district, and national levels.

SUMMARY

In summary, as the athletic trainer continues to venture into the nontraditional, clinical setting, he or she must acknowledge and accept a change in role and responsibility. Although challenging at times, these changes must be viewed as new and positive opportunities. Such opportunities can enable athletic trainers to set the example and serve as role models for other health care professionals. Therefore, the athletic trainer's conduct must reflect a high level of professionalism in order to improve the credibility of the athletic training profession in the clinical setting and to maintain a commitment to excellence.

Study Questions

1. Assume that you are a recent athletic training graduate and have been working with a patient for several weeks now. You have been unable to establish effective lines of communication as he has remained apprehensive and a bit withdrawn. One particular day, however, he "opens up" to you and begins telling jokes. You are delighted that the patient has relaxed and that a looser atmosphere has finally developed. Unfortunately, you notice that a nearby patient has overheard the jokes, many of which were culturally biased, and has been offended. How would you handle this situation?

2. Assume that you are a staff athletic trainer with a few years of experience. One day, your clinic's administrator, also an athletic trainer, calls you into his office and informs you that he is concerned with your lack of involvement in the clinic's programs and activities. He states that you appear to be a "9-to-5'er." Do you interpret this as positive or negative criticism? The administrator proceeds to hand you a copy of a research proposal and asks if you would be interested in leading the investigation. Do you view this as a burden or an opportunity? Explain your answers.

3. You have recently been promoted to sports medicine coordinator of the clinic at which you are employed. One of the staff athletic trainers, with whom you have been friends and colleagues for years, begins wearing extremely tight-fitting skirts and slacks to work. You have had several

male patients comment to you about how appealing they find her new attire. You are quite disturbed by these comments and decide to confront the employee. When confronted, however, she states, "Since there is no established dress code at this clinic and since the patients obviously approve of my appearance, why should I change?" Discuss your reply and possible solutions.

4. You are a staff athletic trainer with several years of experience. Over the years, you have developed a habit of arriving to work late, even if only by a few minutes. Your newly appointed administrator, with fewer years of experience than yourself, confronts you with this matter. She very bluntly states that your tardiness will no longer be tolerated. Explain your initial response and your eventual course(s) of action.

5. Again, assume that you are a staff athletic trainer with a few years of experience. During a treatment session, one of your patients engages you in a conversation about your educational background, innocently stating that she has been informed that you are "just an athletic trainer." Describe your initial reaction and your eventual response(s). How can you handle this situation without destroying your rapport with the patient?

References

1. Reynolds PP. Reaffirming professionalism through the education community. *Ann Intern Med.* 1994;120:609-614.

2. Bryan CS. What is professionalism and can it be measured? (editorial) *JSC Med Assoc.* 1995;91:243-244.

3. Blumenthal D. The vital role of professionalism in health care reform. *Health Aff Millwood.* 1994;1:252-256.

Suggested Readings

Capel S. Attrition of athletic trainers. *J Ath Train.* 1990;25:34-39.

Capel S. Psychological and organizational factors related to burnout in athletic training. *J Ath Train.* 1986;21:322-327.

Cormier J, York A, Domholdt E, Kegerreis S. Athletic trainer utilization in sports medicine clinics. *J Ortho Sports Phys Ther.* 1993;17:36-43.

Knight K. Research in athletic training: a frill or a necessity. (editorial) *J Ath Train.* 1988;23:212.

Krakinowski L. Preventing burnout. *Rehabil Today.* 1992;April:18-23.

Osternig L. Research in athletic training: the missing ingredient. *J Ath Train.* 1988;23:223-225.

Medical History Taking

Gina Lorence Konin, ATC, PT

OBJECTIVES

Upon completion of this chapter, the student will be able to accomplish the following:

1. Understand the importance of obtaining an accurate and detailed medical history

2. Be familiar with questionnaires and pain scales utilized in obtaining a medical history

3. Gain a general understanding of how past or present medical conditions affect the selection of rehabilitative methods

4. Gain an understanding of why it is essential for a clinician to identify medications that a person is presently or has recently taken

5. Identify why the home environment and the type of employment and work-site are important elements in the medical history taking process

Obtaining a thorough and accurate medical history is crucial in providing optimal, safe care. Many nontraditional athletes and patients seen in clinical settings may have very different backgrounds and lifestyles. These varying lifestyles may strongly affect their health status and alter their safety in clinical treatment. Athletic trainers have an extensive background in orthopedic assessment including obtaining an orthopedic medical history. Therefore, this chapter will focus on the importance of medical history taking in the clinical setting as it relates to the nontraditional athlete.

MEDICAL HISTORY

The medical history should include items that may alter the treatment program or items that may modify the expected outcome. Questions specific to the injury are asked in an attempt to identify the location of the pain, the mechanism of the injury, and the time of injury, as well as other pertinent information.

The clinician should devise or follow a format for the medical history taking. A consistent format ensures that the clinician obtains all the necessary and significant information from the patient. It is easy to overlook a question when taking an informal medical history, and such a mistake could be devastating. For example, a clinician might implement an iontophoretic treatment, which involves transferring medication into the body via electricity. The patient may have a reaction to the medication if he or she is allergic to that particular ion. Such a reaction can be avoided by following an organized format for taking a medical history, which could have revealed the patient's allergy.

The clinician should ask open-ended questions to allow the patient to answer as accurately as possible. An appropriate format would be to ask, "does this change your pain in any way?" The questions should not be leading questions such as, "does this make your pain worse?"

The following areas are considered to be essential components of a person's medical history, but by no means are they meant to be all-inclusive.

Pain

Identifying the location of the pain is of clinical importance. The location of the pain may assist in identifying what structure has been injured. For example, medial knee pain may include injury to the medial collateral ligament or medial meniscus. The clinician may ask a patient to "point to where it hurts." It is incumbent upon the clinician to remember that referred pain may not correlate with the actual area of injury.[1] For example, the patient may complain of pain in the lateral brachial region, which may be referred from a glenohumeral joint lesion.[1] It is essential that the clinician inquire if the pain is localized or radiating. Is the pain localized over the lumbar region (possible lumbosacral strain)? Or is the pain radiating? Pain in the L5 dermatome could be from various structures such as the L5 nerve root, the L5 disc, visceral structures with L5 innervation, or from any muscle with L5 innervation.[2]

Pain description may assist with diagnosis. Pain may be described as burning, tingling, sharp, or achy among others. Typically, "pins and needles" sensations may indicate peripheral nerve compression.[1] Reports of a dull ache in the morning are common in degenerative joint disease.[3] Musculoskeletal structures have varying degrees of sensitivity to pain,

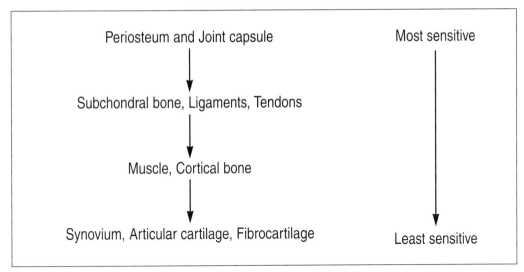

Figure 14-1. The sensitivity of various structural components as a response to noxious stimuli.[1]

while the periosteum and joint capsule are the most sensitive to pain[1] (Figure 14-1).

Pain scales are methods of identifying how a patient perceives his or her pain. There are multiple pain scales utilized today to provide objective ratings for identifying the patients' perception of their pain and to identify changes in their pain. For example, one technique is to have a clinician ask a patient to rate his pain on a scale of 0–10, with 0 being relevant to no pain and 10 indicating the most severe pain imaginable. Another style would be to give the patient a visual analog scale (Figure 14-2a,b).

The visual analog scale is a 10-centimeter long line. The patient is asked to mark the level of perceived pain, in which the distance marked should correlate with the numeric pain scale rating. For example, if the patient rated their pain five on the numeric pain scale then the clinician would expect the patient to intersect the visual analog scale approximately at 5 centimeters or in the middle of the 10-centimeter line.

Another common method used to assess the perception of a patient's pain is the McGill Melzack Pain Questionnaire.[4] This procedure includes not only visual analog scales, but also the incorporation of descriptive words used to describe pain, schematic drawings of the body, and particular questions seeking information about the history of the pain.

Injury

Determining the mechanism of injury provides important data for diagnosing the injury. For example, if the patient reports receiving a blow to the lateral aspect of the knee, the clinician may suspect a medial collateral ligament injury.

It is also important to identify when the injury occurred. Did the pain appear to have an insidious onset and progressively worsen? Many times additional in-depth questions will identify overuse injuries. For example, rotator cuff tendinitis may progressively worsen with overhead activities. This may be seen in carpenters or painters. Acute injuries may be characterized by pain at rest and increased with activity, reports of diffuse pain, and increased skin temperature as a result of recent trauma/bleeding.[5] A chronic injury tends to develop a localized pain with a specific movement but relieves itself with rest.[5]

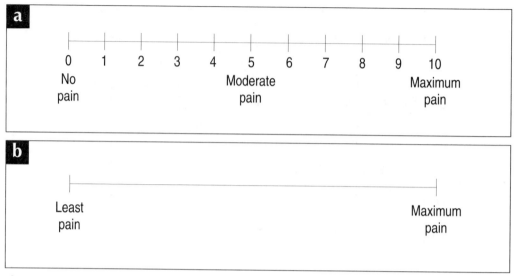

Figure 14-2. Pain Scales demonstrating different methods in which a person can respond as a means of describing perceptions of pain. a) Numeric Pain Scale: the patient is instructed to pick a number that correlates to his or her perceived level of pain. b) Visual Pain Scale: patient draws a line to intersect the horizontal line to indicate his or her perceived level of pain. Typically, the clinician may measure the distance of the patient's intersected line and assess correlation to the numeric pain scale rating.

Age

The patient's age may alter treatment programs or assist in identifying the clinical impression/diagnosis. For example, modalitic interventions are contraindicated in patients with long bone epiphyseal plates that have not closed, which may be seen in adolescents. This situation requires the clinician to choose alternative treatment methods to obtain the optimal outcome. In addition, the patient's age may assist in identifying possible causes of the problem. Osgood Schlatter's disease traditionally develops during an adolescent growth spurt and has a higher incidence in males.[6] By contrast, degenerative diseases tend to occur more frequently in the older population. Osteoporosis is another example of a condition affecting the older population. According to the American Academy of Orthopaedic Surgeons, osteoporosis affects 30% of women over the age of 65 years.[6]

Past Medical History

Events of the past may require program modifications, and the presence of other conditions may affect the patient's response to treatment. Therefore, questions regarding conditions not directly related to the injury should be incorporated. This should include specific questions addressing any presence or history of heart problems, diabetes, cancer, respiratory disorders, or pregnancy. Inquisition should include myocardial infarction, hypertension, and circulatory or pulmonary compromises. See Table 14-1 for a formatted list of classifications. For example, caution is required when applying electrical stimulation to a patient with blood pressure compromises because electrical stimulation may alter blood pressure regulation.[7] In another situation, a patient may be referred for rehabilitation for back pain. Knowledge of a secondary medical problem such as rheumatoid arthritis may

Table 14-1
Secondary Medical Problems that Should Be Considered When Taking a Medical History

- Metabolic deficiencies
- Coronary compromises
- Respiratory compromises
- Vascular compromises
- Dermatologic conditions
- Neurological deficits

modify the time of day for optimal treatment. Rheumatoid arthritis patients tend to loosen up later in the day and may tolerate exercise better in the afternoon. By contrast, a patient with osteoarthritis may have less pain in the morning because the joints have not yet been aggravated as a result of daily compressive and shear forces.[8] Patients with asthma tend to tolerate exercise better in a warm, humid environment and with gradual increase in workouts.[9] Refer to Chapter 18 for a more detailed look at conditions regarding nonorthopedic pathologies. These disorders require greater awareness in response to treatment and may require avoidance of various modalities because of the body's decreased ability to safely respond to such methods of treatment.

Pregnancy requires special consideration. Multiple treatment approaches for injuries in this population are unsafe. Electrical stimulation is contraindicated during pregnancy.[10] Pregnancy creates hormonal and chemical changes within the body, and these changes may affect orthopedic injury healing or may increase the risk of injury as a result of increased ligamentous laxity.[11] It is recommended that pregnant women follow cautious guidelines during exercise including maintaining a maternal heart rate below 140 beats per minute, avoiding supine exercise beyond the fourth month of gestation, and limiting strenuous exercise to 15 minutes.[12]

Discussion of previous treatment or previous surgeries may assist the clinician in several aspects. The clinician may opt to try a previous treatment that was successful if the present injury is similar to the past injury. The clinician may prefer to devise a new program if the previous treatment was unsuccessful. This needs to be determined on an individual basis because the success of previous treatment methods depend on many factors, including patient compliancy and clinician skills.

Previous surgeries may limit present outcomes. Multiple or previous surgeries create trauma to the area which results in swelling, pain, and possible fibrosis among others. The patient may not have attained full range of motion or strength from previous surgery. The clinician should consider this when devising expected goals and outcomes.

Medications

This is another extremely important aspect of the medical history. Medications may mask the patient's perception of pain.[3] Medications may also alter sensory input.[13] Therefore, using pain as a guideline may not be safe. Medications may also alter the heart's response to exercise. Beta blockers tend to lower the maximum heart rate during heavy exercise, as rates rarely exceed 120 beats per minute.[14] The clinician may need to frequently monitor heart rate and blood pressure during treatment with the understanding that medications may modulate responses.

Medications may effect the rate of healing. Corticosteroids impair wound healing.[15] Long-term use of corticosteroids may cause general tissue edema, thin, fragile skin, collagen tissue weakening, increased pain threshold, proximal muscle weakness, and osteoporosis.[3]

Patients may be allergic to assorted medications or topical agents. The clinician should inquire about possible allergies or allergic reactions to medications (previous cortisone injections, aspirin or prescription medications, topical over the counter creams) Clinicians utilize lotions, gels, and medications to apply ultrasound, massage, iontophoresis, or phonophoresis. Safety is a concern at all times and the clinician may risk harm if unsure of a patient's allergies. Therefore, an inquiry to drug allergies should be made to prevent complications. For a more thorough understanding of pharmacological interaction in rehabilitation, the reader is referred to Chapter 19.

Lifestyle

Active people tend to have a better fitness level as compared to sedentary people. Regular exercise may increase the cardiovascular functional capacity and may decrease myocardial demand for oxygen during physical activity.[16] Lifestyle may alter the severity and healing response of an injury. For example, smoking increases the blood pressure and high blood pressure increases the pressure on the arteries, increasing the potentiality for rupture of the vessels.[17] High fat diets increase the probability of build up along the vessels.[17] Constriction of blood flow may slow healing of injuries. The patient is also at a higher risk for a myocardial infarction or a stroke if the lifestyle includes smoking, lack of exercise, increased blood pressure, increased serum cholesterol, or obesity.[18] A person's lifestyle is always a consideration in returning the patient to pre-injury status.

Home Environment

Recognizing the home environment helps define the rehabilitation program. A person who has undergone a total knee replacement may have multiple stairs to climb to get to the kitchen. Therapeutic exercises should include quadriceps and hamstring strengthening, step-ups, and others. Another case scenario involves a person who has incurred an ankle sprain and as a result has poor balance or proprioception. Identifying and recommending removal of throw rugs in the home may prevent re-injury or additional injury.

Employment

The understanding of a person's occupation should be implemented into the treatment program. If a person lifts 20-pound cases for 8 hours each day, then the final stages of rehabilitation should include strengthening exercises, multiple lifting exercises to simulate the work place, and instruction in lifting mechanics to prevent re-injury. The rehabilitation program may include a graduated progression of resistance, repetitions, and postural positions to simulate the return to work. Frequently the injured worker undergoes a functional capacity assessment prior to returning to work. This assessment is similar to a functional test for an athlete prior to returning to sport. The functional capacity assessment may last up to 4 or 8 hours and consists of functional tasks: sitting, standing, walking, numerous material handling lifts, and a validity section. This data is collected and reviewed to determine safe guidelines for the injured worker to return to work.

Those that spend most of the day sitting at a desk may benefit from postural training and a work space analysis, in addition to indicated treatment programs. A work space analysis may be performed to identify changes in the office that may prevent re-injury or aggravation of the injury. The market offers numerous devices to limit musculoskeletal strain, especially in the office environment. Examples of work-site modifications include changing the desk height to decrease cervical or lumbar strain, using a lumbar roll in the office chair to provide lumbar support, and changing the angle of a computer keyboard to possibly alleviate carpal tunnel irritation. Knowledge of the patient's employment requirements and job-site are critical components necessary to achieve optimal rehabilitative, restorative levels.

Patient Goals

Patient goals are possibly the most important and overlooked consideration in the rehabilitation process. What does the patient want or expect to gain from rehabilitation? Following an ACL reconstruction, the patient may simply want to gain enough knee motion to drive his or her car independently and walk up and down one flight of stairs normally. These goals must be considered. The clinician can avoid frustration by learning this early in the rehabilitation process as opposed to trying to convince a person that he or she must complete potentially difficult and unnecessary tasks. For example, a successful 15-minute run on the treadmill at 8 miles per hour as a criteria to be discharged may not be required for someone who has no desire to perform such activities upon completion of rehabilitation.

Questionnaires or scales may be completed by the patient to assist with gathering information. Written forms may be more helpful for the patient in terms of remembering items when he or she sees them listed. (See example form in Figure 14-3.) The clinician could give the patients such forms prior to the initial evaluation or first visit. Otherwise the clinician should read through the forms together with the patient to ensure desired responses. Ample time should be allotted for questions and discussion of the forms.

SUMMARY

The medical history taking is a vital component in providing optimal, safe care. In taking a medical history, the clinician should ask open-ended questions to allow the patient to answer as accurately as possible. These questions should include information about the following categories: pain, injury, age, past medical history, medications, lifestyle, home environment, employment, and patient goals. The past medical history should specifically address the presence of metabolic deficiencies, coronary, respiratory, or vascular compromises, dermatology conditions, and neurological deficits, among others. The clinician may utilize various forms to assist in gathering information such as a functional rating form or pain scales.

Study Questions

1. List and describe the components of a medical history as discussed in this chapter.
2. Discuss the importance of obtaining an accurate and thorough medical history.

Activity

_____   I have normal use of this injured area. I can do everything including strenuous sports and/or heavy labor.

_____   I can perform strenuous activities but at a lower level than before.

_____   No recreational activities are possible.

_____   Daily activities are difficult and cause persistent symptoms, but they can be done.

_____   Daily activities cause severe problems and are rarely attempted.

Check the following activities that are painful or difficult:

_____   combing hair   _____   reaching a top shelf

_____   brushing teeth   _____   going up or down steps

_____   putting on a shirt   _____   driving an automobile

_____   tying or putting on shoes _____   grocery shopping

Explain why the above activities are difficult
(e.g., limited motion, pain, weakness.)

_____

_____

I can sit _____ minutes consecutively.

I can walk _____ (minutes or miles) maximum.

Figure 14-3. Functional Rating Form.

3. Describe a visual analog pain scale. Include a drawing.
4. Devise a medical history questionnaire.
5. Discuss why a clinician should identify medications that a person is taking while under the care of an athletic trainer.
6. Discuss why information regarding lifestyle may be valuable information gathered in the medical history.

References

1. Lynch MK, Kessler RM. Pain. In: Hertling D, Kessler RM, eds. *Management of Common Musculoskeletal Disorders: Physical Therapy Principles and Methods.* 2nd ed. Philadelphia, Pa: JB Lippincott; 1990:40-59.

2. Magee DJ. *Orthopedic Physical Assessment.* 2nd ed. Philadelphia, Pa: W.B. Saunders; 1992.

3. Hertling D, Kessler RM. Assessment of musculoskeletal disorders. In: *Management of Common Musculoskeletal Disorders: Physical Therapy Principles and Methods.* 2nd ed. Philadelphia, Pa: JB Lippincott; 1990:60-80.

4. Melzack R. The McGill Pain Questionnaire: major properties and scoring methods. *Pain.* 1975;1:277-299.

5. Kessler RM. Concepts of management. In: Hertling D, Kessler RM, eds. *Management of Common Musculoskeletal Disorders: Physical Therapy Principles and Methods.* 2nd ed. Philadelphia, Pa: JB Lippincott;1990:81-86.

6. American Academy of Orthopaedic Surgeons. *Athletic Training and Sports Medicine.* 2nd ed. Park Ridge, Ill: Author; 1991.

7. Kloth L. Interference current. In: Nelson RM, Currier DP, eds. *Clinical Electrotherapy.* Norwalk, Conn: Appleton-Century-Crofts; 1987:183-207.

8. Samples, P. Exercise encouraged for people with arthritis. *Physician and Sports Medicine.* 1990;18:123-127.

9. Stamford, B. Exercise-induced asthma: Taking the wheeze out of your workout. *Physician and Sports Medicine.* 1991;19:139-140.

10. Newton R. High-voltage pulsed galvanic stimulation: Theoretical bases and clinical application. In: Nelson RM, Currier DP, eds. *Clinical Electrotherapy.* Norwalk, Conn: Appleton-Century-Crofts;1987:165-182.

11. Eisenberg A, Murkoff HE, Hathaway SE. *What to Expect When You're Expecting.* New York, NY: Workman Publishing Co.; 1991.

12. Morales K, Inlander CB. *Take this Book to the Obstetrician with You: A Consumer's Guide to Pregnancy and Birth.* Addison-Wesley Publishing Co.; 1991.

13. Jackson-Klykken O. Brain function, aging, and dementia. In: Umphred DA, ed. *Neurological Rehabilitation.* St. Louis, Mo: CV Mosby; 1985.

14. Herbert WG, Froelicher V. Exercise tests for coronary and asymptomatic patients: Interpretation and exercise prescription. *Physician and Sports Medicine.* 1991;19:129-133.

15. Moncur C, Williams HJ. Rheumatoid arthritis: Status of drug therapies. *Phys Ther.* 1995;75:511-525.

16. American Heart Association. *Healthcare Provider's Manual for Basic Life Support.* Dallas, Texas: Author; 1988.

17. American National Red Cross. *Standard First Aid.* St. Louis, Mo: Mosby Lifeline; 1993.

18. O'Sullivan SB. Coronary artery disease. In: O'Sullivan SB, Schmitz TJ, eds. *Physical Rehabilitation: Assessment and Treatment.* 2nd ed. Philadelphia, Pa: FA Davis Co.; 1988:307-334.

CHAPTER
15

Clinical Documentation

Chris Arrigo, MS, PT, ATC

OBJECTIVES

Upon the completion of this chapter, the student will be able to accomplish the following:

1. Identify the purposes of effective documentation

2. List and describe the four major types of writing styles

3. Describe the essential criteria for rehabilitation providers as standardized by Medicare

4. Better understand the importance of appropriately organizing medical documentation in a clear, concise, and consistent manner

The documentation of findings in the medical record is one of the most important and most overlooked areas of clinical athletic training. Today's medicolegal climate necessitates both the careful and systematic documentation of objective findings and functional measures of progress to determine the appropriateness of the interventions rendered to any client. The clinician must remember that often the determination of payment and judgment of effective treatment practices is made by a third party that may have a limited knowledge of the actual practice of rehabilitative services. Because the payment for health care by a third party is the customary method of reimbursement for services rendered to a client, successful communication in the medical record is imperative. An effective system of documentation must therefore gather and record pertinent information concerning every client, including subjective comments and measurable objective and functional findings, as well as provide a clinical assessment and a treatment plan for every client. The purpose of effective documentation also serves to 1) assess quality assurance, 2) assess treatment outcomes, 3) communicate with other professionals, 4) provide organizational structure, and 5) standardize procedures.

WRITING STYLES

The type of writing styles one chooses can play an important role in patient care as well as achieving success with third party reimbursement. To be complete with documentation, one needs to be complete, thorough, and organized in the presentation of the subject's record. It is important to remember that you as the clinician may be the only person to actually physically treat an individual. Therefore, it becomes your sole responsibility to be able to "tell the story" to others in a convincing and believable manner. This can be accomplished regardless of the style of writing one chooses.

While many styles of writing exist, some are more common than others. With respect to therapeutic documentation, the most common writing styles are 1) narrative, 2) problem-oriented, 3) anecdotal, and 4) S.O.A.P. note format. The process by which one chooses one style over another can be determined by a number of factors. These factors include but are not limited to individual preference, educational background, facility policy, and type of clinical setting. Regardless of the type of style chosen, appropriate information must still be included to assure complete documentation.

The *narrative style* most directly tells a story. The information concerning a client is presented in complete sentences and paragraphs. Initial assessments, progress notes, and discharge notes often include this style of writing. The advantage of this is that it follows the standard style of reading, thus providing for a clear summary of relevant information. The major disadvantage is that one does need to read through paragraphs to pick out specific points of interest with respect to each client, as opposed to looking at individual tables and data that might reveal other interesting findings. While narrative documentation can be extremely thorough, longer reports of client information tend to pose a challenge for the reader when looking for relevant information.

The *problem-oriented style* of medical documentation uses a format by which each client problem is enumerated and all entries concerning each problem are grouped together in separate categories. This style of documentation is most often utilized in facilities where various clinicians are all documenting about the same group of problems on a client.

The advantages of this system lie in the ability to coordinate services of multiple disciplines around a focused problem list for each and every client. The disadvantages range from the complicated nature of this style of writing to increased time and content constraints on the clinician. This type of documentation is most often utilized in a hospital or multidiscipline rehabilitation facility.

The *anecdotal style* of medical documentation necessitates the use of preprinted forms. With these forms minimal writing is required by the clinician and only pertinent information concerning a client is recorded in blanks. The anecdotal style allows for essential material to be recorded quickly; however, the development of the forms is time consuming and costly. Although information can be obtained easily from these forms, often material not included on the forms is not recorded.

In the *S.O.A.P. note format* of documentation, information is recorded as it pertains to four categories: subjective (S), objective (O), assessment (A), and plan (P). Subjective information is any and all information gained from sources other than clinical measures. Most often information about an injury or condition is derived from the client as well as from other sources, such as coaches and families. In the objective category, tests and measures, undisputed facts, and unbiased observation concerning a client are recorded. The assessment portion of the medical record is the clinician's professional opinion regarding the disposition of findings and progress of the client. The final portion, the plan, is an outline of the treatment techniques and interventions to be implemented to manage the problems that have been identified.

The three biggest advantages of the S.O.A.P. note format are 1) information is logically organized, 2) it does not depend on grammatical correctness, and 3) it can be completed quickly. However, the disadvantages include the fact that the reader must be familiar with the profession and the normal course of treatment to completely understand this documentation format.

MEDICAL RECORD ORGANIZATION

The client's chart or medical record is the official source of all medical, legal, and financial information. This information must be properly organized and presented in a way that meets the standards of third party payers. If all of the information required is not contained within the client's chart, then typically payment will be denied. A lack of documentation, regardless of any treatment rendered, reflects an absence of care. The most important considerations in the standardization of documentation are the consistency of entries (either typed or handwritten), forms utilized, placement, and identification, as well as forms completed in a reasonable time period.

All guidelines for third party reimbursement are based on an organized presentation of the information obtained and recorded concerning a client. The criteria that outlines this information can be found in the Standards of Practice of the American Physical Therapy Association, the Medicare system rules and regulations, the law, and individual insurance provider requirements. Each of these entities has particular documentation standards, all of which may vary slightly. We will present the most common and accepted documentation standards and practices, but clinicians are encouraged to investigate specific implications as they relate to their geographic location and type of clinical practice.

Table 15-1
APTA Standards of Practice

Initial Evaluation

Medical history
Diagnosis
Problem list
Complications and precautions
Physical status and limitations
Functional status and limitations
Critical behavioral, mental, social, and
  environmental factors
Goal list
Clinical assessment

Plan of Care

Treatment interventions
Frequency
Duration
Coordination of care
Client/family involvement
Anticipated status at discharge

Progress Note

Change in status
Appropriate supervision
Follows established plan of care
Client progress

Discharge Planning

Social/environmental needs
Outside referrals
Community resources
Recommended follow-up
Outcome related to initial evaluation
Disposition

Table 15-1 presents an outline of the American Physical Therapy Association's Standards of Practice for Physical Therapists. These standards reflect the physical therapy profession's opinion of the minimum content of documentation recommended to reflect quality of clinical care in a rehabilitation setting.

Clinical Documentation Standards

The documentation standards that have the greatest overall effect on third party reimbursement and the clinical practice of rehabilitation in any setting are those of the Medicare program. However, clinical athletic trainers have very little direct contact with Medicare clients. Because Medicare is the largest third party payer with some of the strictest documentation guidelines, it makes most other insurance carriers and regulatory agencies adopt standards similar to those imposed by Medicare. Thus, a thorough understanding of the Medicare documentation standards is essential in the athletic training arena.

Medicare standards outline the following four essential criteria for rehabilitation providers, all of which must be included in client documentation for services to be considered complete and, therefore, reimbursable:

1. Medical necessity
2. Skilled care
3. Significant progress
4. Reasonable intensity

Rehabilitative services must be *medically necessary*, in that all services must be considered an accepted effective medical practice for the injury, surgery, or condition of the client.

The necessity for *skilled care* in the services rendered is the second criteria that must be met. In physical therapy documentation this refers to the fact that the services rendered to a client must be complex and sophisticated enough that they only can be performed by or under the supervision of a physical therapist. The same requirement should hold true for any professional and thus athletic training services should also meet the same standard.

The expectation of *significant progress* refers to the requirement that the physician and clinician expect that the condition will improve considerably in a reasonable and relatively predictable period of time.

Reasonable intensity is the amount, frequency, and duration of rehabilitative services rendered for the condition for which the client is being treated. In clinical athletic training, reasonable intensity may require significant justification above and beyond general comments; for example, twice or three times a day for 6 or 7 days per week may be reasonable. The specific reasons and functional justifications to ensure speedy and safe return to competitive athletics must be outlined completely to support this type of reasonable intensity.

Medicare regulations also include six documentation criteria required of the rehabilitation provider. These criteria are outlined in Table 15-2. The absence of any of these criteria from the client record can render even eligible care unreimbursable.

Although a referral or physician's prescription is a common document in all ancillary practices, Medicare regulations require all of the specific information outlined in Table 15-2 within the physician's script. If this information is not contained in the referral then it must be contained within the initial evaluation and plan of care. The referral should contain the diagnosis requiring athletic training services and the services desired. Request for these services can be worded in general terms (e.g., evaluate and treat) or specific terms (e.g., post ACL-PTG rehabilitation program).

The initial evaluation should be performed routinely the first time a clinician sees a client. This document and any subsequent re-evaluations must record baseline subjective and objective data as it relates to the client's status and functional limitations. It should, therefore, demonstrate the need for skilled rehabilitative services. At a minimum, the initial evaluation should contain relevant medical history and the client's subjective comments regarding his or her condition, an assessment of pain and chief complaint, loss of functional status, range of motion, muscular strength and power, proprioceptive and coordination measures, neurovascular status, stability and special tests, as well as determination of endurance or cardiopulmonary function.

All information should be recorded objectively in acceptable units of measure, including the following:

1. Information regarding a client's **pain** should be recorded in two forms: a) on an analog pain scale that ranges from 0–10, and b) how it affects function in the client (e.g., pain prevents an athlete from throwing a baseball over 50% of his normal capacity).
2. **Functional limitations** should be recorded in how they affect normal daily activities and athletic participation. For example, in lower extremity and spine pathologies this should include how the condition affects walking, climbing stairs, squatting, doing activities on uneven surfaces, kneeling, lifting, and running. Upper extremity functional levels should be described in relation to how an individual can function with his arm away from his body and overhead, and lifting capacity along with a

---

Table 15-2
Medicare Documentation Criteria

Physician Referral

Diagnosis
Significant past history
Current medical findings
Physician's orders
Goals, if determined
Contraindications
Rehabilitation prognosis
Client's awareness of diagnosis
Previous rehabilitation

Initial Evaluation

Baseline data of client status that demonstrates the need for services performed by the clinician. This document should include, as appropriate, the following:
    Loss of mobility
    Loss of limb
    Self-care capability
    Pain
    Range of motion
    Strength
    Endurance
    Cardiopulmonary function
    Coordination
    Posture
    Wound status

Plan of Care

Problems identified
Treatment goals
Treatment interventions
Medical necessity of care
Physician signature
Frequency
Duration

Daily Documentation

Date
Treatment
Change of status

Progress Note

Care received
Skilled supervision of care
Progress made toward goals
Changes in status
Changes in treatment plan
Response to treatment

Discharge Summary

Treatment received
Progress made during treatment
Total treatments received
Disposition
Prognosis

---

description of limitations in sporting activities.

3. **Range of motion** can be recorded in either the degrees of motion present in a plane or by the percentage of normal range of motion present. For example, range of motion can be expressed as 90° of shoulder abduction and/or 50% of the normal range of motion. Recording the percentage of motion present often is beneficial to nonspecialty reviewers of third-party claims.

4. **Muscular strength and power** can be recorded using manual muscle testing techniques or isokinetic performance testing, and/or relating deficits to the performance of functional activities. Again, the recording of this information in terms of a percentage of the normal range provides a clear description of the client's deficits.

5. **Proprioception and coordination** can be expressed by measures ranging from simple descriptions of a single leg Rhomberg balance test or scapulohumeral rhythm to complex computer-driven balance and coordination testing.

6. Documentation of **neurovascular status** simply requires the appropriate use of dermatome sensation assessment, reflexes, and vascular tests as required by the

---

Table 15-3
Hints for Writing Good Documentation

1. Write legibly, clearly, and concisely.

2. Use few abbreviations. Explain sports medicine terminology when appropriate.

3. Report range of motion and muscle strength/performance as a percentage of normal, in addition to degrees and muscle grade.

4. Use one standard documentation format that includes all necessary information.

5. Rely heavily on objective measures and functional activities.

6. Progress should be expressed in functional terms. These terms include daily activity, athletic, and/or job requirements. These terms will vary from client to client.

7. Document what the client *cannot* do rather than what he or she *can* do.

8. Do not try to fool an insurance reviewer. Fraud is a crime.

9. When in doubt on setting frequency and duration of treatment, utilize physiologic healing parameters as a guide.

10. Do not overtreat.

11. Use black ink only.

12. All errors should be corrected with a single line through the error and initialed and dated next to the line. No scribbles or white out should be used.

13. If a standardized rehabilitation protocol is referred to, a copy should be included in the medical record for reference.

---

client's condition.

7. The status of **joint stability** and other special tests related to the specific pathology or condition being evaluated should be recorded also.

8. **Cardiopulmonary or muscular endurance** should be presented as it relates to the individuals capacity to perform activities in relation to time and intensity as compared to pre-injury or normal expected functional performance.

Although this list is not all-inclusive, all additional evaluation tests and measures should be documented in a similar fashion (Table 15-3).

Following the recording of the subjective and objective baseline information, the clinician should make an assessment of the client and his or her condition as it relates to the need for skilled rehabilitative interventions. This should include the formulation of a list of problems based on the information gathered previously. For each problem identified during an evaluation, a corresponding goal should be developed to solve or improve the problems identified. The clinician also should provide his or her clinical impression and prognosis for the attainment of the goals outlined in the assessment portion of the evaluation. The predicted frequency and duration of treatment, along with the types of interventions to be utilized during treatment, should all be outlined in the plan portion of the note. All documentation should be signed by the clinician in legible script or with a printed/typed name as it appears on his or her license under the signature.

The plan of care should be included as a portion of the initial evaluation. Many agencies and reviewers require it to be a separate form. The separate form is easier to modify and can be communicated back and forth between the referring physician and clinician for review and signature, and it can also serve as the certification of care document. Normally an updated care plan is required every 60 days following the initial evaluation. The care plan should include a list of the problems identified during the initial evaluation, all of the interventions or treatment measures that will be utilized to address the problems, and a list of goals that these interventions will be designed to obtain. The goals listed should be outlined in both pathokinesiological terms and functional parameters. For example, a goal for a 50% quadriceps strength deficit could be worded as: "the goal is to increase strength of the right quadriceps by 50% to allow for unrestricted running, cutting, and functional athletic activities that currently cannot be performed independently." The expected frequency and duration of treatment should also be included within the plan of care. The expected course of treatment should be reasonable for the medical condition of the client and be in line with the normal course of physiologic healing times and the expected prognosis for the specific diagnosis.

This document also should contain a statement of medical necessity for the skilled care to be rendered. This type of statement is crucial for reimbursement and can be worded along these lines: "The client requires skilled athletic training services to address the problems and achieve the goals outlined within the plan of care. Rehabilitation potential for this client is good. The client tolerated the initial evaluation and treatment (with or without) problems or difficulties, and exhibits good knowledge and understanding of the treatment program outlined. The problems, goals, and treatment plan were discussed with the client and the client agrees."

Each treatment session, or daily note, should contain at a minimum: the date, current subjective comments and/or changes in the client's condition, two to three key objective markers for continual comparison with previous measures, the treatment and interventions rendered, any change in status and description of treatment tolerance, and an outline of the plan for changes or advancement on the next visit. This information should be concluded with the clinician's signature.

Progress Notes

Progress notes frequently are defined in two varying ways by medical reviewers. One is as an expanded treatment note and the other as a weekly summary note of client progress. These notes simply serve to summarize progress made over small intervals of time, usually once a week or every 2 weeks.

Using the S.O.A.P. note format, a progress note should contain specific comments regarding the condition (subjective); treatment received—client response/progress (objective), progress made toward established goals—goals achieved; changes in previous treatment plan and goals (assessment); course of treatment over next time period—discharge planning activities (plan).

Progress and discharge summaries are formal summations of the care a client has received over a specific period of time, normally 30 days. This type of documentation is used to demonstrate the coordination of care rendered to a client and to summarize all progress made in the reporting period. This format is critical to demonstrate progress that is frequently not identified in daily documentation. This type of summary typically coincides with a re-evaluation of the client. Notations in this form of documentation should include a summary of the type of treatments received, progress made within each problem area, total number of treatments received, as well as all changes in the current plan of care, or the final prognosis and disposition of the client if the note is a discharge summary.

The following is an example of a narrative format of a progress summary, as described by Brown:

Dear Dr. (name),

(Client name) was initially evaluated on (date) for the treatment of (diagnosis/condition, should include left/right side if applicable).

Treatment has consisted of (actual treatment rendered) for (duration and frequency of treatment). During this time, (client name) has (response to treatment). This is based on (objective and functional findings). (Client name) reports (any subjective statements).

The plan at this time will be (treatment plan, goals to be addressed). The prognosis for (client name) is (professional opinion of ability to attain goals).

OUTCOME MANAGEMENT IN DOCUMENTATION

Clinicians must continue to develop their practices by demonstrating the efficacy and efficiency of their treatment approaches. Clinicians must be able to demonstrate that what they do is effective both in rehabilitating our clients and in holding down costs. The documentation requirements and standards outlined within this chapter will continually be enforced with greater zeal by every third-party administrator. The trend today is directed toward making clinicians responsible for their practice patterns—one of the many examples directed toward addressing rehabilitative costs in the practice of confining therapy to less than 10 visits for the vast majority of acute musculoskeletal conditions.

Third-party payers continue to take the initiative in attempting to control rehabilitative costs by many methods, including computerized auditing of claims, fee schedule reimbursement, increased peer review, case management, increased fraud investigation, hiring of medical personnel for claims review, selective provider contracting, and discount fee negotiations. All of these things indicate that the burden of proof regarding the necessity of care now falls squarely on the clinician. Payers are demanding proof of treatment efficiency and cost-effectiveness.

Clinicians must strive to be as objective as possible in all measures reported and define limitations and problems, along with their matching goals, in functional terms. The key to good documentation is linking the objective impairments identified within the evaluation to the client's inability to function and perform activities.

SUMMARY

Clinicians must be able to measure deficits related to their client's physical condition, appropriately document those measures, and finally relate them to functional problems and goals that can be sequentially monitored and repeatedly assessed. The ability to demonstrate progress in a reasonable period of time based on the pathology involved is imperative to effective documentation. The guidelines presented within this chapter are minimum standards and key indicators necessary to meet these challenges in today's clinical environment.

Study Questions

1. What is the importance of effective documentation with respect to the profession of athletic training?
2. Explain the differences between narrative, problem-oriented, anecdotal, and S.O.A.P. note writing styles. What are the advantages and disadvantages of each?
3. Using the S.O.A.P. note format, document a treatment session for an athlete to whom you recently provided athletic training services.
4. Explain how documentation standards play a role in third party reimbursement for athletic trainers. Why should an athletic trainer be familiar with those guidelines set forth by Medicare?
5. The plan of care should always include a list of goals for the client. Devise a list of both short- and long-term goals for an athlete who has recently sustained a second degree medial collateral sprain to his left knee. Be sure to include temporal and measurable components in your goals.
6. With the following sentence that has been recorded in a narrative style note, explain how you would make a correction to change the active range of motion from 75 degrees to 85 degrees: "Post rehabilitation measurements revealed an increase in shoulder flexion AROM to 75 degrees."

Suggested Readings

Griffith J, Ignatavicius D. *The Writer's Handbook: The Complete Guide to Clinical Documentation, Professional Writing and Research Papers.* Baltimore, Md: Resource Applications Inc; 1986.

Kane RA, Kane RL. *Assessing the Elderly: A Practical Guide to Measurement.* Lexington, Mass: DC Health & Company; 1981.

Kettenbach G. *Writing S.O.A.P. Notes.* Philadelphia, Pa: F. A. Davis Co; 1990.

Logan C, Rice KM. *Medical and Scientific Abbreviations.* Philadelphia, Pa: J. B. Lippincott Co; 1987.

Medicare Provider Notice 96-20. *Special Instructions for Documentation.* Washington, DC: September 4, 1996.

Walter JB, Pardee GP, Molbo DM. *Dynamics of Problem-Oriented Approaches: Patient Care and Documentation.* Philadelphia, Pa: J. B. Lippincott Co; 1976.

Special Considerations for Industrial Athletic Training

Martin R. Daniel, MS, ATC

OBJECTIVES

Upon completion of this chapter, the student will be able to accomplish the following:

1. Identify the similarities and differences between the nontraditional industrial, nontraditional clinical, and traditional athletic training settings

2. Describe the appearance of a typical patient treated in the industrial athletic training setting

3. List and describe the specific educational needs that are associated with industrial athletic training

4. Identify the components essential for administering an effective industrial athletic training program

As the year 2000 approaches, more and more athletic trainers are exploring the industrial athletic training setting. This environment is not clearly defined; however, it typically consists of a corporation, company, or group of employees whose main function of employment is not of the athletic or sporting nature. This is not to say that athletic or physical attributes are not needed to complete the tasks at hand. Instead, it simply means that the population of people who are treated in the industrial setting hold positions that are not based on wins and losses.

There are many factors that must be weighed by those contemplating a career in the industrial nontraditional settings of athletic training. Therefore, clinicians and educators have a responsibility to properly prepare those who wish to pursue a career in this arena. When the founders of the NATA listed the disciplines by which all athletic trainers practice, they were casting a template that would carry the organization beyond the traditional athletic training room. Basic principles of issues such as case management, utilization review, injury prevention, the study of injury cycles, and capitation of services were just a few areas that were targeted. These principles have been taught and revised for over 50 years by the NATA and athletic trainers. And today other health care systems of the world are listening to this time-tested programmatic approach.

Employment in an industrial athletic training setting poses many differences from that of the training room, and even the typical clinical outpatient type setting. This chapter will focus on some of the unique features found to be essential for a person to successfully work in the industrial athletic training setting: patient population, special educational needs, and specific management requirements.

PATIENT POPULATION

The typical patient that an athletic trainer may find in an industrial setting can range in age from the late teens to 65 years and older. Again, unlike the traditional athlete, those who may be treated in an industrial setting will present with varying degrees and levels of health status, motivation, and attitude. In addition, the trainer may be faced with the workers who act under the jurisdiction of a union, and thus may need to meet special requirements prior to returning to full performance of duty (Figure 16-1).

These differences place the athletic trainer in a more involved position by the way of a health educator and a resource provider. Topics of guidance may range from injury management to general fitness and health concerns, and require the athletic trainer to place special emphasis on motivational needs of patients.

Because of the varying presentation of patient profiles, the athletic trainer must also possess patience and flexibility when assessing the appropriate rehabilitation guidelines for each individual. It is known from experiences with well-trained athletes that individuals heal at different rates. This situation may become exaggerated when dealing with nonathletic, generally sedentary individuals. Even if treatment regimens are rigidly adhered to, not all clients may achieve success during the rehabilitation process.

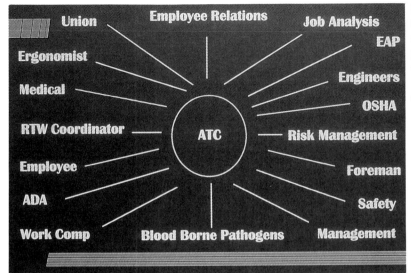

Figure 16-1. A representation of the many departments and disciplines that an athletic trainer working in an industrial setting may encounter.

SPECIAL EDUCATIONAL NEEDS

The Surgeon General's Report on Health Promotion and Disease Prevention in 1979 adopted the Canadian Health Fields Model (CHFM) as a useful concept for identifying the elements that contribute to death and disease. In this report, four major elements were identified:

1. Environmental hazards
2. Human biological factors
3. Behavioral factors or unhealthy lifestyles
4. Inadequacies in the existing health care and ancillary systems

When applied to problems of occupational health, the health field model emphasizes that an individual's illness or injury is the result of several occupational and nonoccupational influences, and that these influences may differ from person to person. These elements can also be applied to work-related musculoskeletal injuries. However, it becomes important to emphasize that some of the components provide the opportunity to be addressed through preventative measures.

Environmental Hazards

Hazards to the musculoskeletal system associated with work are described as work place or work-site traumatogens. A traumatogen is defined as a source of biochemical stress stemming from job-related demands that exceed the worker's strength or endurance. Examples may occur during episodes of heavy lifting, repetitive actions, or forceful manual twisting. Traumatogens can be measured by determining the frequency, magnitude, and direction of forces that are required to complete a task and comparing these forces to a person's posture and the points of application of these forces.

Human Biological Factors

Human biological factors refer to the genetic ability or natural characteristics that influence a worker's capacity for safely performing a job. Examples may include the worker's physical size, strength, available range of motion, work endurance, and the integrity of the musculoskeletal system. These are some of the primary factors that account for variability in performance capability in the industrial population and the potential mismatching of an individual worker with a particular job. Hence when job demands habitually exceed the worker's capabilities as defined by such physical attributes, the health and safety of the worker become compromised.

Behavioral Factors or Unhealthy Lifestyles

The element of an unhealthy lifestyle as a result of a behavioral factor refers to acquired behaviors or personal habits that may increase a worker's risk of incurring musculoskeletal strain or injury. Such behavioral factors may include insufficient sleep or recovery from exertion, the perception of a job as being excessively demanding or hazardous, job dissatisfaction, or mental lapses due to response interference. Lifestyle factors can more specifically include obesity, lack of adequate physical fitness, poor dietary habits, and substance abuse. Recent studies have also focused on personality factors that may be predictive of permanent disability.

Inadequacies in the Existing Health Care and Ancillary System

A concern that always exists within any work-site or industry is a lack of medical knowledge and appropriate training for health care personnel with regard to etiology and management of musculoskeletal injuries that result from biomechanical strain. Management, design engineers, and workers require special health and safety training in order to become familiar with traumatogens and to recognize the role of biological and behavioral risk factors as they relate to musculoskeletal injuries. Such people would also benefit from training in the principles of prevention and health promotion.[1]

Failure to attend to the needs of workers with disabilities creates a cost to society in a number of ways. First, severe financial implications may impact an industry as a result of labor turnover and additional recruitment. Second, additional effects on work force participation for those who must complete the tasks of the workers with disabilities must be considered. In addition, few workers are active to sustain systems of social insurance and benefits from financial contributions.[2]

Business and industry have come to realize that healthy employees can help reduce costs. Many industrial firms have reassessed the practice of simply "pensioning off" chronically injured or disabled employees. Instead, they have realized that experienced employees represent an investment, an appreciating asset, and a resource to their firms. Goldfarb suggests that America's competitiveness in the world market depends, to an extent, on the industry's ability to keep workers healthy, fit, and on the job.[3]

Not only does an employer have an investment in an employee in the areas of training costs, work experience, and goodwill, but a healthy employee is more productive, may be less prone to accidents, take fewer sick days, and use fewer health insurance benefits. Soon after assuming the position of President of the Chrysler Corporation, Lee Iacocca discovered that Blue Cross/Blue Shield was the company's biggest supplier. Chrysler was spending more money on health care than for steel and rubber.[4] Chrysler is not the only company that has been faced with such a situation.

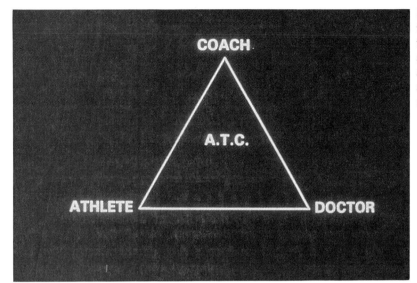

Figure 16-2a. The relationship of an athletic trainer with a coach, an athlete, and a physician as seen in the traditional athletic training environment.

Cost-containment of worker's compensation medical expenses has become the focus of heightened discussion among many disciplines. Standard industry practice has been to send an injured employee either back to work, home, or to an outside doctor or hospital for treatment and rehabilitation. The extent of controlling the levels of treatment and rehabilitation then lies outside of the hands of the individual company.[5]

Over the last 50 years, the NATA and certified athletic trainers have provided all of the previously mentioned programs. In the earlier years, however, these programs were made available only to those who were competing in athletics. Today, there are numerous other groups and organizations that can benefit from the expertise of an athletic trainer. As athletic training continues to expand into the industrial environment, it will be necessary to develop and be proficient in plant safety, ergonomics, and work station analysis programs. These are areas that are not exclusively addressed by any one profession. Yet the addition of athletic trainers to the industrial medicine team may provide for increases in overall employer production and decreases in expenses.

Most medium to large industries have staff proficiency in plant safety, but having some background in this area helps the athletic trainer to better integrate the prevention and rehabilitation programs to occupational safety considerations. However, not all plant safety personnel are proficient in ergonomics. Because the process of designing an ergonomically correct job station involves an analysis of both body mechanics and job requirements, athletic trainers working in an industrial setting should seek further education in the area of ergonomics.

ADMINISTERING AN INDUSTRIAL ATHLETIC TRAINING PROGRAM

When working in the industrial setting, a person often feels like that round peg that is being wrenched, pounded, and often sandwiched into that square hole. The industrial setting does have its own unique characteristics when dealing with day-to-day operations. This is the time when it becomes most important for a clinician to remember his or her

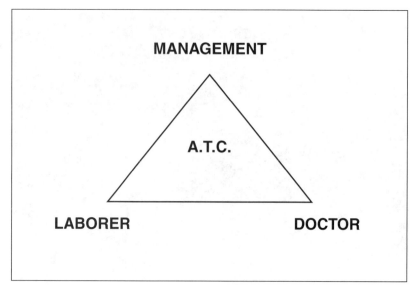

Figure 16-2b. The relationship of an athletic trainer with management, an employee (laborer), and a physician as seen in the industrial athletic training environment.

roots and foundation as an athletic trainer. The model depicted in Figure 16-2a demonstrates how an athletic trainer works within a traditional setting. The same model with some modification can also be used within the industrial setting (Figure 16-2b). Working as a liaison between the athlete, coach, and attending physician can be compared to working with an employee, manager, and an attending physician.

The formula for success has already been established by athletic trainers for some time now. Nobody can guarantee that the transition from a traditional athletic training room environment to an industrial setting can be an easy one, but an individual can always apply those principles previously learned to help him or her succeed during a transitional phase. For example, every time a new head coach is hired at a university, administrative processes usually change and all of those must adapt to the surrounding environment. In the industrial setting, the head coach is the management, thus it becomes that person's responsibility to communicate and adapt with his or her personnel.

The industrial setting also has other similarities to the traditional athletic training room; for example, team members' names and faces remain relatively constant. In fact, industry turnover rate may be slightly smaller than that of an athletic team, thus promoting long-term case management capabilities.

When 70%–80% of all injuries in the industrial setting fall within the categories of strains, sprains, contusions, and first aid, it becomes easy to recognize the value of the athletic trainer as an asset to industry. These figures are echoed in the state of Michigan, according to the Michigan Occupational Safety and Health Administration (MIOSHA), as seen in Figures 16-3a and 16-3b.

Athletic trainers have used these figures to demonstrate their needs in the industrial settings. As in other cases, marketing of a person's qualifications and services are an essential component to creating more positions for potential employment.

Once the education of the employees, union, and management staffs has been completed, the process of providing injury rehabilitation as well as fitness and conditioning programs to the employees can begin. Programs should be designed to decrease the number of days lost due to work-related injuries—a similar goal when dealing with athletes.

The study of ergonomics and work station analysis should then be implemented. This

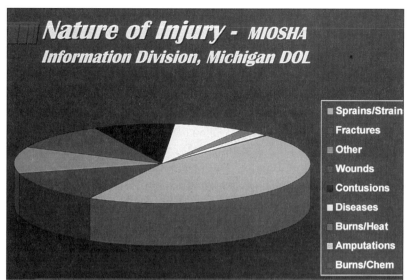

Figure 16-3a. Breakdown of the nature of injuries seen in industrial settings as reported by the Michigan Occupational Safety and Health Administration (MIOSHA).

Nature of Injury - MIOSHA
Information Division, Michigan DOL

- Sprains/Strain
- Fractures
- Other
- Wounds
- Contusions
- Diseases
- Burns/Heat
- Amputations
- Burns/Chem

Figure 16-3b. Breakdown of the nature of injuries seen as reported by the Occupational Safety and Health Administration.

Nature of Injury - OSHA

Sprains/Strains	45 %
Fractures	12.8%
Other	10.8%
Wounds	10.5%
Contusions	8.8%
Occ. Diseases	7.3%
Burns/Heat	2.1%
Amputations	1.2%
Burns/Chemical	.4%

is accomplished by first educating yourself, and then those around you. Providing regularly scheduled safety education meetings, work-site analysis, and assessing job performance levels may all contribute to the overall goals of the industrial athletic training program. A key to success when designing and implementing this type of a program is remembering that the treatment of athletes and employees possesses many similarities, yet also many differences. Knowing when to apply various approaches and techniques may make the difference between a successful and an unsuccessful industrial program.

One should always recognize that sensitive issues may arise, and that athletic trainers in the industrial setting are not immune to personnel challenges. Establishing client population and working to meet the needs of both the injured employee and management may be a difficult task. A trainer's first alliance should always be to take care of the injured individual—this will usually prevent potential conflicts. In some cases, an employee and his or her union may view the athletic trainer and program as a part of management. This can be a serious threat to the trainer's existence in the industrial setting. If the trainer is not trusted by his or her employees (his or her team), then they may not seek the trainer for services. The art of being a successful athletic trainer has always been in maintaining rapport and integrity with team members and colleagues. The proper development of preventative and rehabilitative policies that clearly outline employee and employer benefits will go far in cultivating both client and union respect.

The athletic trainer needs to remember the primary reason for his or her existence in the industrial setting. Essentially, the athletic trainer is no different than any other assembly line employee. Although the medical staff, the employees, and even the union may be impressed with the trainer's abilities, qualifications, and the results of the program, he or she still has an obligation to management. That obligation is to effectively document and support cost-effectiveness to the company. The best way for the athletic trainer to do this is to closely observe and collect data with respect to the number of working days lost by an employer as a result of an injury and the insurance premiums or other additional health care costs that may have been reduced since being with the company. An athletic trainer should be careful to use the number of reported injuries as a reason for his or her necessity, because the mere existence of the trainer may lead employees to seek medical attention for a given condition when, in fact, they may not have done so previously.

Management may expect the trainer to collaborate with them to establish criteria in the areas of eligibility for services, treatment and coverage of work-related versus non-work-related conditions, preventative programs, emergency procedures, and record keeping among other issues that relate to the position.

Administratively, it will be imperative to maintain the following:
1. Supervision and facility upkeep
2. Security provisions of all records, reports, and related materials
3. An implemented public relations campaign
4. Quarterly and annual personnel of staff on site
5. Delegation of responsibilities for daily operations of the facility
6. Sound procedures as approved by the medical director

SUMMARY

The industrial athletic training setting exhibits many similar characteristics to that of the traditional athletic training room setting. The primary difference lies in the age, varying levels of health, varying levels of motivation, and associated needs of the task at hand. Like the traditional setting, an athletic trainer must continue to become educated in his or her surrounding as well as being able to educate those around him- or herself in order to provide for optimal atmospheres. This especially holds true in the industrial setting, because successful ventures may continue to lead to the proliferation of career opportunities.

Athletic trainers planning to establish a career in the industrial setting must become familiar with topics such as ergonomics, occupational health and safety, labor relations, worker's compensation, environmental disease and industrial hygiene, work-site wellness, work simulation and conditioning, functional capacity testing, cost justification, budgeting, and human resource management.

Study Questions

1. Describe the differences between the industrial athletic training setting and those previously discussed in this text.
2. What type of modifications does an athletic trainer working in an industrial setting need to make to achieve success with a preventative and rehabilitative program?
3. Specifically what type of behavioral factors may lead to an increase in work-related injuries or illnesses? Can these be modified?
4. As an industrial athletic trainer working for a large corporation, what would be your primary goals when administering an injury program? What components or programs would you need to consider to accomplish these goals?
5. How could you as an athletic trainer realistically implement occupational safety programs in an industrial company with approximately 2,000 employees?
6. What type of data or factual information would you need to support your validation of being hired as an athletic trainer in an industrial setting?

References

1. U.S. Department of Health and Human Services. Proposed National Strategy for the Prevention of Musculoskeletal Injuries. DHHS (NIOSH) Publication No. 89-129.
2. Galvin D. Health promotion, disability management and rehabilitation in the workplace. *Rehabilitation Literature*. 1986;47:218-223.
3. Goldfarb H. An insider's guide to choosing rehabilitation. *Risk Management*. 1989;36:46-50.
4. Moretz S. Chrysler takes a new look at in-plant medical care. *Occupational Health*. 1989;51:39-41.
5. Major M. The industrial athlete. *Safety and Health*. 1990;4:64-67.

CHAPTER 17

Special Considerations for the Nontraditional Athlete

Larry Gardner, ATC, LAT, PT

OBJECTIVES

Upon the completion of this chapter, the student will be able to accomplish the following:

1. Identify the role of the athletic trainer when working with nontraditional athletes

2. List the behavioral and physical characteristics of rodeo athletes

3. Identify common treatment procedures involved in rodeo events

4. Recognize those nontraditional athletes involved in motor sports

5. Appreciate the nature of injuries seen and common treatment methods for motor sport athletes

Aparadigm shift is necessary for athletic trainers who enter the realm of treating "nontraditional" athletes. Although the athletic trainer may consider a sport or an athlete "nontraditional," the athlete certainly feels that his or her sport is as traditional as any other sport. As previously mentioned, classifying a prototype nontraditional athlete may be difficult. In an attempt to give yet another viewpoint of how one should prepare for and care for nontraditional athletes, this chapter will take a look at two very different, nontraditional, yet ever-growing popular sports and those who participate in them. The sports and groups of athletes that will be addressed here are the participants in rodeo and motor sports.

Rodeo skills were being developed long before the first American football, baseball, or basketball games were ever practiced or played. The first car race probably took place not long after the first two horseless carriages appeared in the same town or on the same road. The point being that while there are sports not routinely or adequately covered by athletic trainers, these sports are considered as traditional as mom and apple pie to those involved.

The athletic training profession must continue to take strides to have a definite objective of athletic training coverage for any and all sports where there is a danger of the competitors being injured. Athletic training curricula should provide education and exposure to ensure that athletic trainers are prepared to cover sporting events of all types in an attempt to provide the care that the participating athletes deserve. While this process begins in the classroom, it is the sole responsibility of the individual athletic trainer to broaden his or her expertise through continuing education and clinical experience, because it may not be feasible for him or her to gain experience in all areas during academia. As with the industrial athletic trainer, preparation and validation may be the key to creating larger numbers of jobs in these nontraditional areas.

RODEO

One of the most recent groups of athletes that has come under the care of the athletic trainer is the rodeo cowboy. There are a number of reasons for the rodeo athlete's late arrival to the scene of athletic training. While some athletic trainers who work the rodeo circuit may have the luxury of a training room, more often than not a trailer, tent, or the back of a pickup truck serves as a substitute (Figure 17-1).

The nomadic lifestyle of the rodeo athlete is an obstacle in providing the necessary care that is needed on a regular or scheduled basis. A cowboy or cowgirl may be entered in five rodeos per week, each in five different cities and states. In order to offer any level of consistent care for this group of athletes, the ability to move the needed equipment and/or personnel at the same pace or to the same locations is imperative.

Yet another obstacle for the rodeo athlete is the fact that historically the natural and expected thing to do if one is injured is to "cowboy up"! To cowboy up in the rodeo world is to take care of yourself, expect no help, do the best you can on your own, and continue to "get on" or compete.

A mistake made in the medical field for years was to treat the cowboy as any other person would be treated, i.e., to have him or her stop doing whatever causes the injury, possibly immobilize the involved area, or tell him or her, "you can't do that anymore." The

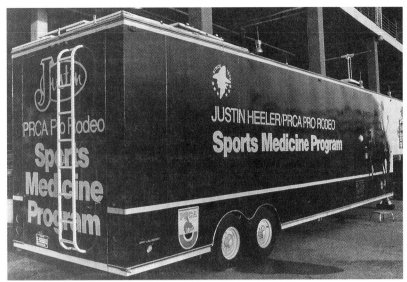

Figure 17-1. A truck bed that has been converted to a mobile athletic training room for the pro rodeo. Although this is very beneficial, it is not the norm for most rodeo events.

early decision makers in sports medicine did not understand that a rodeo athlete pays an entry fee to have the opportunity to compete, and must actually physically compete to have any chance of winning money or getting paid. In fact, a cowboy can compete, make his or her ride, score well, and still make no money. There is no injured reserve or salary protection in the rodeo. The rodeo cowboy or cowgirl lost faith in the medical practitioners who failed to realize that the athlete is going to compete if at all possible and sometimes even when they consider it impossible.

Many times an athletic trainer's responsibility is to protect the rodeo athlete in the best possible manner and to the highest degree possible because the athlete is going to do whatever he or she wishes to do whether the athletic trainer feels as though he or she should compete or not. This places the athletic trainer in a precarious position. However, it is one he or she must accept while protecting the rodeo athlete to the highest degree possible under the circumstances. In all circumstances, the trainer should always document decisions, treatments, and recommendations as a means of formality and protection.

Remember that while a 200-pound football player may be asked to compete against an opponent that outweighs him by 75 pounds or even 100 pounds, in reality the 175-pound rodeo cowboy is asked to compete against a 1,500–2,000-pound competitor. Because of this tremendous difference in weight as well as strength, the injury incidence is very high (Figures 17-2a through 17-3).

Treatment of Rodeo Athletes

Covering rodeo events offers an athletic trainer the opportunity to exercise his or her knowledge of the field of athletic training to a greater extent than in any other sport. Preventive and restorative techniques are taught on a regular basis in an attempt to allow the rodeo athlete to foster a sense of independence with respect to his or her own health maintenance (Figure 17-4).

Teaching the rodeo cowboy the importance of stretching to prevent injury is very beneficial to the cowboy and rewarding to the athletic trainer. Twenty years ago seeing a rodeo cowboy stretching before his or her event was extremely rare. Today the chute area at a

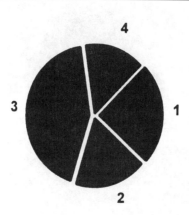

Figure 17-2a. Rodeo injury statistics by specialty.

1 -- 24% compete in bareback riding.
2 -- 18% compete in saddle bronc riding.
3 -- 43% compete in bull riding.
4 -- 15% compete in various timed events.

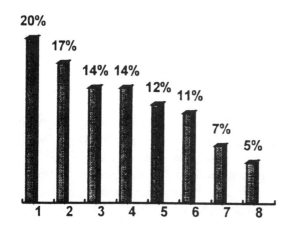

Figure 17-2b. Rodeo injury statistics by anatomy.

1 -- 20% are various spine injuries.
2 -- 17% are hand, wrist and elbow injuries.
3 -- 14% are knee injuries.
4 -- 14% are foot, ankle or leg injuries.
5 -- 12% are groin and hamstring injuries.
6 -- 11% are shoulder injuries.
7 -- 7% are miscellaneous injuries
8 -- 5% are head and face injuries.

Saddle Bronc Riding
1. Knee (constant flexing of joint)
2. Lumbar / Lower back
3. Shoulder
4. Thigh / Groin
5. Ankle

Bareback Riding
1. Elbow (forceful hyper extension)
2. Lumbar
3. Hand
4. Wrist / Shoulder (tie)

Bull Riding
1. Thigh / Groin (rider small relative to bull's back)
2. Knee
3. Shoulder
4. Elbow
5. Head / Face

Calf Roping
1. Thigh / Groin (stepping off horse)
2. Lumbar / Knee (tie)
4. Shoulder / Ankle (tie)

Steer Wrestling
1. Knee
2. Ankle
3. Shoulder (arm rotated to grasp horn)
4. Lumbar
5. Cervical Spine

Bullfighting
1. Knee (ligament injuries)
2. Lumbar
3. Ankle
4. Lower Leg
5. Thigh / Groin

Figure 17-2c. Rodeo injury statistics by event.

rodeo could easily be mistaken for a warmup area for the ballet.

Teaching the rodeo cowboy how to preventively apply athletic tape to him- or herself is of utmost importance because adequate athletic training coverage at events may be absent at 80%–90% of rodeos each year. There is no other athlete that has learned to fend for him- or herself as much as the rodeo cowboy, through necessity. Most bareback riders and bull riders can probably tape their own elbow as well or better than many athletic trainers. Many bull riders and bullfighters can tape their injured knee with the best of athletic trainers. This is a tribute to the athletic trainers who have taught them to do so and a tribute to the rodeo cowboys for the ability to accept the fact that there will not always be someone there to take complete care of them.

Most events involved with rodeo last no longer than 8 seconds. Yet it is essential to be able to convince a cowboy that the nature of his or her demanding schedule requires not only strength training but also proper conditioning in the form of aerobic conditioning. Endurance has become a key component to a cowboy's success.

Teaching this athlete the importance of proper nutrition is also important. Because of the nomadic lifestyle, constant travel, and time constraints, the ability to maintain a healthy diet becomes quite difficult. Education is the key, and these athletes tend to be very receptive to and appreciative of any sound advice.

The athletic trainer's first aid and initial care for injury skills are called upon in rodeo more so than in any other sport. Traumatic injury is commonplace when competitors are asked to compete with adversaries that outweigh them by ten-fold. It becomes our responsibility to be prepared to be called upon often for the administration of first aid treatment, and to also explain to the participants the importance of properly caring for acute incidents when appropriate medical personnel are not immediately available.

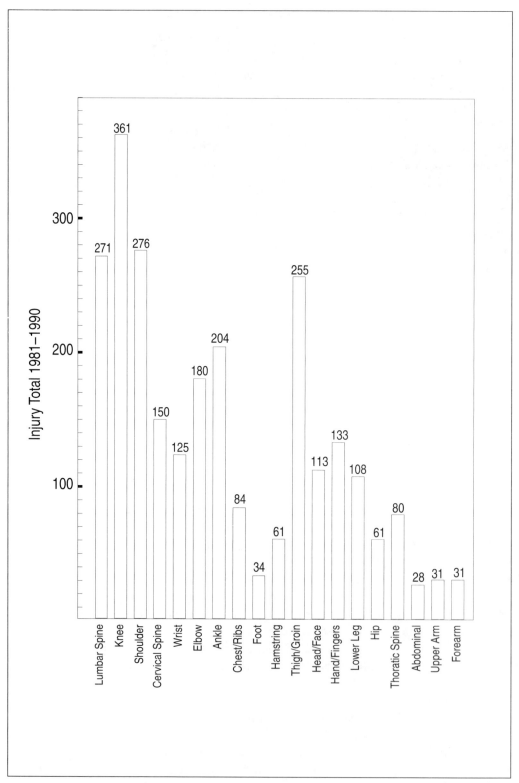

Figure 17-3. Professional Rodeo Circuit Association (PRCA) injury report by anatomical location.

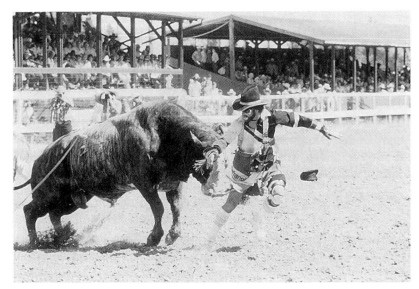

Figure 17-4. Treating injuries at a rodeo provides the athletic trainer with a unique approach to athletic care.

Although the concept of "PRICE" (protection, rest, ice, compression, elevation) is often followed, the resting part is a difficult concept for the rodeo athlete to follow. Because athletes may be on the go in preparation for an upcoming event, it may be necessary to treat them on the go and teach them to properly care for themselves.

Rehabilitation is also a very important area in which the athletic trainer can provide instruction. Very few rodeo athletes have the privilege to attend supervised rehabilitation programs on a regular or extended basis. Again, the ability to convey simple, yet effective exercise techniques that a cowboy can take with him or her will be of much benefit. When covering rodeo events on a regular basis, it makes sense to have exercise or first aid handouts explaining follow-up care for some of the more common injuries that may be encountered by the athletes.

As with other sports that encounter physical contact, and possibly more so with the rodeo, the athletic trainer must be prepared to face and react correctly to life-threatening situations. The danger that is involved with this sport must clearly be recognized and helped. Team preparation, to also include emergency medical technicians and physicians, is imperative. As in all other sports, "who" does "what" should be established prior to the beginning of any performance or event.

MOTOR SPORTS

Race car drivers and their team members travel constantly throughout the sports year. They are, like many athletes, required to participate in their sport or job when they are not at 100% of their physical capabilities. The athletic trainer is again placed in the position of being called upon to assist an athlete to compete during a time of injury. When dealing with this group of athletes, the athletic trainer must be prepared to accept this challenge.

During the course of working with motor sports, an athletic trainer may find him- or herself spending more time caring for the support staff of a driver than the driver. The pit crew is placed under tremendous pressures, and they work with very technical, expensive,

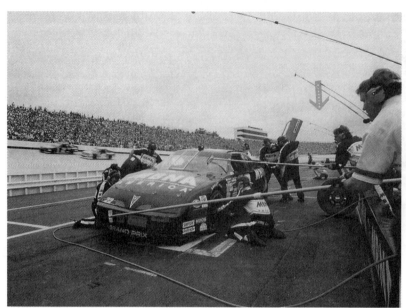

Figure 17-5. Although a motor sport driver is resting during a pit stop, he is unable to adequately adjust his posture. Meanwhile pit crew members are working quickly and efficiently to ensure a smooth transition. Photo courtesy of Dover Downs.

flammable, and unforgiving equipment. Time spent in "pit stops" has often been the difference between a driver winning and losing a race. It therefore becomes imperative that the crew is able to function efficiently and quickly. This task must be accomplished whether a person is injured or not (Figure 17-5).

The athletic trainer who finds him- or herself covering motor sports may not often deal with a driver who is injured during a race. Unfortunately, because of the severity and danger of many wrecks, emergency medical personnel are required to be on hand at all times. These professionals are responsible for transporting drivers who have experienced traumatic injuries. Typically, ambulances are utilized and the injured driver is taken either to the on-site track hospital or infirmary, or transported via helicopter to a designated hospital.

Interaction between the athletic trainer and the driver involved in a wreck would more commonly occur during the rehabilitation process depending on the nature of the injury. This may include treatment sessions, instruction in the application of preventive taping and protective padding, or simply assistance with flexibility exercises. The most common areas of injury that athletic trainers are called upon to care for deal with the spine (49%), the lower extremity (28%), and the upper extremity (23%).

Teaching the motor sport athletes the basic principles of prevention, treatment of acute injuries, and nutrition should be objectives for an athletic trainer involved with this type of activity on a regular basis.

Education regarding injury prevention is also a vital component when working with drivers. These individuals spend long periods of time in a seated, cramped position with minimal movement of either their upper or lower extremities. Correct stretching and postural training may aid in the prevention of the development of abnormal body mechanics and potential injury.

Aerobic conditioning may be beneficial to both the driver and the crew members. The driver must perform with extremely quick reflexes over multiple repetitions for essentially hours at a time. The crew members, however, must work very long hours during the race week and race day, and then work very quickly and efficiently during pit stops regardless of when they might occur during the race. It is important to remember that the driver and crew members must work quickly and efficiently not only to determine who wins and who loses, but sometimes to distinguish between life and death.

Nutritional education also has a role in motor sports. Many times these athletes are called upon to work in varying circumstances. Changes in eating habits, regular exercise, and even temperature can lead to adverse bodily conditions.

The administration of athletic first aid is common during race week, especially to the support staff (pit crew). The most common injured areas that the athletic trainer will treat with respect to the support staff in motor sports include the spine (66%), the lower extremity (17%), and the upper extremity (17%).

Having the knowledge to correctly treat themselves for those injuries is very important to a driver and pit crew members. They may be able to obtain treatment at times during their busy schedule and lifestyle, but more often than not they will not have that privilege. Therefore, the athletic trainer who can teach them to care for themselves will be providing a tremendously valuable service.

SUMMARY

Whether dealing with the nontraditional athletes or settings that have been discussed in this chapter or anywhere else, it is the responsibility of the athletic trainer to prepare him- or herself in order to provide knowledgeable services in otherwise unfamiliar arenas. There is the need to understand not only the athletes themselves, but also to have a working knowledge of that particular sport or event to ensure that good, sound decisions can be made.

Many times an athletic trainer may be placed in a situation where the athlete makes a decision to continue to compete against the athletic trainer's recommendation. In such a case, the athletic trainer must protect the athlete to the highest degree possible. The athletic trainer should also protect him- or herself by documenting the given recommendation and the athlete's decision to disregard the recommendation. Athletic trainers must always remember the responsibility to the athlete, but never forget the responsibility to themselves and their family.

Study Questions

1. Explain how an athletic trainer would design a preventive exercise program for a rodeo athlete. Repeat for a motor sport athlete.
2. How can an athletic trainer successfully prepare to cover a rodeo event? What are the essential components that a trainer should possess in order to be adequately prepared?
3. What specific types of injuries might an athletic trainer expect to find when dealing with motor sport drivers? What about with pit crew members?
4. Suppose you have provided acute care to a rodeo cowboy who you believe has just torn the ulnar collateral ligament of his thumb. You do not

believe that he should continue in his next and final event, even though he is a finalist in the competition. However, the cowboy disregards your recommendation and decides to compete anyway. How would you handle this situation?

Suggested Readings

ATCs Treat Rodeo Cowboys. *NATA News*. March 1992:15.

Owsley HK. The traveling training room. *NATA News*. June 1994:12-13.

Riley R, Carey GB. Eating on the road. *NATA News*. December 1994:18-19.

Recognition of Nonorthopedic Medical Pathology

Jeff G. Konin, MEd, ATC, MPT
Ron Courson, ATC, PT, NREMT
Hank Wright, ATC, PT

OBJECTIVES

Upon completion of this chapter, the student will be able to accomplish the following:

1. Recognize the importance of nonorthopedic-related medical pathology as it relates to treating the person as a whole

2. Become familiar with common conditions of the immune, endocrine, nervous, respiratory, cardiovascular, circulatory, and integumentary systems

3. Become familiar with the relationship of malnutrition and the healing of orthopedic injuries

4. Become familiar with common diseases of the blood

5. Recognize the implications for athletic trainers with respect to common nonorthopedic related pathology

The field of athletic training is unique, with the certified athletic trainer (ATC) serving in a variety of roles, ranging from the prevention of injuries to emergency management to evaluation, treatment, and rehabilitation, with supervised progression and return to functional activity. The athletic trainer of today has evolved into an allied health professional, whose practice is based on scientific principles and physiologic rationales. Because of the very nature of athletics itself, the ATC is exposed to a variety of orthopedic-related injuries. In fact, in many athletic training settings orthopedic injuries may constitute the majority of pathologies encountered. However, the ATC must always be cognizant of the possibility of nonorthopedic medical pathology. The purpose of this chapter is to discuss recognition of nonorthopedic-related medical conditions, provide an overview of common pathology, and consider the influence of nonorthopedic pathology on performance.

The rapidly evolving clinical athletic training setting has additionally created an increased emphasis on education regarding nonorthopedic medical pathology. The clinical athletic trainer may serve a more diverse population versus the traditional setting athletic trainer, with a wide range of ages and backgrounds. An increased interest in health and fitness has created a new population of physically active individuals. Likewise, an increase in athletic activities for people with disabilities has created a new population of athletes and athletic-related injuries. These new areas, and the increased potential for exposure to nonorthopedic pathology, underscore the importance for the ATC to be well-versed in pathophysiology, having an awareness of diseases and the relationship between the disease process and clinical illness.

The ATC often serves as an initial evaluator and, in this role, must facilitate medical care by recognizing signs and symptoms and referring to the appropriate health care provider(s). This chapter should remind the ATC to have a high index of suspicion and be aware of "red flags," which may indicate important pathology. The old adage, "you see what you look for, you recognize what you know" should also remind the ATC of the importance of education in this area. The ATC should take care in all situations to look at the total picture, to take a comprehensive patient history, and to conduct a thorough physical examination, utilizing the problem-solving approach to assess patient pathology. In contrast to orthopedic pathology, general medical problems may in many instances be less than obvious and only picked up by the well-trained clinician.

A brief overview of nonorthopedic medical pathology follows. This is by no means intended to be a comprehensive listing, but simply an introduction to a system review of various pathologies that may impact the clinical athletic trainer during the decision-making process. For a more comprehensive review of nonorthopedic medical pathology, the reader is referred to the Suggested Readings at the conclusion of this chapter.

IMMUNE SYSTEM

Human Immunodeficiency Virus (HIV)

The human immunodeficiency virus (HIV) is recognized as the causative agent for the disease commonly known as acquired immune deficiency syndrome (AIDS). People who have contracted HIV possess a deteriorating immune system that leads the person to become much more susceptible to infections and illnesses. Although few people die of the virus itself, the disease is terminal and secondary illnesses will eventually overcome a person's ability to fight them off.[1]

The process by which the virus works is by attacking white blood cells in the body that are primarily used to fight off infection and disease. It can be transmitted through the blood as well as in the semen, and is believed to be most transferable via direct contact of mucous membrane structures within the body. Researchers believe that the virus can only enter the body through an opening, as opposed to penetrating through intact skin surfaces. These openings may consist of natural areas such as the mouth, vagina, penis, and rectum, or may include open wounds or any breaks in the skin.

The time frame between when one contracts HIV to the actual period of development of AIDS varies. This period, referred to as the latent period, typically ranges from 2 to 8 years. The importance of recognizing this long latent period lies in the fact that many physically active patients may actually be carrying the virus without even knowing it. Therefore, an athletic trainer must follow all universal precautions with each and every patient, especially when dealing with open wounds of any kind.

Recognizing and identifying a patient who is carrying HIV is not an easy task. Symptoms may include rapid or slow uncontrolled weight loss, fever, diarrhea, and generalized weakness, among others. The conditions will typically worsen in the later stages, when one may experience neurological changes such as dementia and confusion.

Implications for Athletic Trainers

As the number of persons contracting HIV is rapidly increasing at alarming rates, it is incumbent upon the athletic trainer to be aware not only of symptoms associated with the virus, but also how a physically active individual with HIV can continue to participate in daily activities with appropriate modifications. Controlling the sterility of the environment is key because a person's immune system may not be functioning at its highest level. Also, the level of cardiovascular conditioning may play a role in the type of exercise that may be performed. The ATC should always remember that not all people infected with HIV are in the later stages of AIDS or are unable to perform independent tasks. Many, in fact, continue to participate in high level competitive sports. Of utmost importance is to remember that these individuals are still human beings, and that their dignity should be respected at all times.

HIV does not discriminate. All are susceptible to acquiring this condition. It was previously thought that this was a disease that only presented itself in the homosexual and intravenous drug abuser populations. This is no longer the case. Many well-documented cases have demonstrated that promiscuous heterosexuals as well as others have acquired this virus. As an athletic trainer, you should always protect yourself when dealing with patients who present with open wounds. The reader is referred to Appendix D, the NATA's position statement on blood-borne pathogens, for further information on protection of open wounds.

DIGESTIVE SYSTEM

Malnutrition

Athletic trainers have been taught well about the importance of counseling athletes on nutritional concerns as they relate to optimal performance. In the traditional setting, conditions such as anorexia nervosa and bulimia are not uncommon findings among athletes.[2] Although the clinical setting is not exempt from these conditions, nutritional deficiencies often seen in the clinical environment may differ slightly from those in the collegiate and high school environment.

The importance of proper nutrition and its relationship to physiological measures such as increasing blood circulation, facilitating healing of tissue, and removing waste products from injured sites cannot be under-emphasized in any population. It has been mentioned previously that perhaps one of the main components that differentiates the clinical athletic trainer from his or her counterparts is that of the age of the person whom he or she is treating. The age of the physically active is increasing at rapid rates. The clinical athletic trainer must recognize the circumstances under which the older, physically active person may be modifying dietary intake, thus interfering with physical performance and possibly recovery from injury or illness.[3]

There are a number of reasons why an individual may alter his or her nutritional status. Often injury alone forces a person to restrict the type of foods that can be ingested. For example, a person with diabetes may not be allowed to eat many foods with high sugar content. In addition, a person who has recently undergone medical tests or surgery for internal discomfort or illness may have a difficult time digesting certain foods, and therefore be unable to receive the recommended daily allowances of vitamins and minerals. This type of information can be discovered during the process of taking a thorough medical history.

The clinical athletic trainer may find him- or herself working with individuals who are faced with tremendous financial constraints.[4] The reasons of financial difficulty may range from a number of outstanding bills to a decreased income as a result of entering the retirement years. It is not uncommon to find out that these individuals are not properly taking care of their bodies with respect to dietary intake. Typically, these individuals will eat less desirable foods, or even eat smaller amounts of food during each meal, as a method of saving money. Because this may be a common practice for many, it becomes more of a concern if it interferes with a person's ability to heal at desirable rates. The recognition of slower healing as a result of malnutrition is also a difficult situation to identify.

Implications for Athletic Trainers

Identifying states of malnutrition may play an important role in the facilitation of healing. The changes in health care have resulted in sending patients to the clinical settings at much earlier times than was previously done. In the past, patients were kept in acute care facilities until they were completely stabilized and well on their way to recovery. Today, in an effort to increase savings, hospitals are no longer keeping patients in their facilities for extended stays unless absolutely necessary. This means that those in need of rehabilitation services are arriving at out-patient facilities in more fragile stages of health. It therefore becomes crucial that the athletic trainer and the entire rehabilitation team recognize any condition that may deter a person from improving his or her medical status. Not picking up on nutritional deficiencies may eventually lead to longer rehabilitation stints and thus prolong supervised care.

To no one's surprise, communication is the key to understanding a person's nutritional lifestyle. A common finding among those being treated in a clinical setting is a complaint of gastrointestinal discomfort. For example, a patient may report that he is not eating well, if at all, due to the discomfort that he is experiencing. Symptoms also may include dysphagia, vomiting, and diarrhea.

Inquiry into the situation may frequently reveal that this discomfort is simply a result of the medication that the patient is currently taking for the said condition. Simply instructing the patient to report this side effect to the physician can lead to a different prescription for a similar acting medication from a different pharmacological family, thus alleviating previous gastrointestinal discomfort. This, in turn, may allow the patient to return to normal eating habits, and eventually help with the recovery of an injury or illness.

Asking the athletic trainer to specifically identify the type of nutritional deficiency that may exist in an individual that has manifested itself in prolonged treatment may be unfair. This is where the athletic trainer has an opportunity to utilize other team members. In this instance, a recommendation for a referral to a nutritionist or a consult with the patient's physician is very appropriate. Regardless, proper intervention not only improves the condition at hand, but may also prevent future illnesses or diseases from arising.

ENDOCRINE SYSTEM

Diabetes Mellitus

Taking care of the diabetic athlete is not new to the athletic trainer. In fact, many athletes who compete with diabetes are very much aware how to care for themselves in a way that in fact educates many athletic trainers. In the clinical setting, however, different levels of motivational self-caring may be seen among various patients. These individuals are often faced with orthopedic pathology that must be treated and cared for. Therefore, the ATC should be aware of the unique treatment approaches and considerations that an individual should follow when dealing with orthopedic injuries for a patient who has an underlying diabetic condition.

Diabetes mellitus is a condition whereby the body has an inability either to produce insulin or to distribute insulin in sufficient quantities. Generally, three factors play a key role in creating a homeostatic environment for the diabetic: diet, exercise and insulin. Clinically, the person who has diabetes mellitus can be defined as either being insulin dependent or non-insulin dependent. Insulin dependent diabetes mellitus (IDDM) is also referred to as type 1 diabetes and requires the injection of insulin to regulate carbohydrate metabolism. Non-insulin dependent diabetes mellitus (NIDDM) individuals have the potential and ability to control carbohydrate metabolism by means of properly balancing diet and exercise.

When the process of controlling carbohydrate metabolism is poorly followed, one of two circumstances may arise. First, it is possible that the body can build up an abnormally high level of carbohydrates that are not being taken up by the distribution of insulin. This condition, commonly referred to as *hyperglycemia*, can lead to a state called a "diabetic coma." In this instance, an individual over time will develop feelings of lethargy and dehydration. A classic "fruity breath" may be noted as a result of increased acidosis.

Because exercise has the ability to use carbohydrate stores from the body, one must replace these stores regularly to maintain adequate carbohydrate balances. If these sugars are not replaced, one may be left with excessive insulin that is unable to be taken up by carbohydrate sources. This condition of *hypoglycemia*, can lead to a more severe condition called "insulin shock." Symptoms of insulin shock have been described as hunger, nervousness, trembling, irritability and convulsions. The person may eventually perspire, feel light-headed and lose consciousness.

Implications for Athletic Trainers

At times, recognizing the difference in symptoms from a diabetic coma and insulin shock may be unclear. The clinical athletic trainer should make every effort to understand a patient's history if in fact he or she is diabetic. On each visit, conversation and communication should consist of the patient's current state of maintaining carbohydrate balance. This enables the athletic trainer to predict the level of exercise that should be prescribed for the treatment that day. It also may indicate whether or not the patient needs to supplement his or her system with carbohydrates or insulin prior to any exercise session.

Medically, the treatment for diabetic coma is to return to balanced states by injecting doses of insulin. By contrast, insulin shock can be reversed by taking in quantities of carbohydrates. However, when the ATC has a difficult time determining whether a patient is in a state of insulin shock or a diabetic coma, the choice of treatment tends to be that of assuming the patient is in insulin shock. Therefore, when in doubt, increase the person's sugar intake. The addition of sugar to a patient in insulin shock could turn out to be life saving. Whereas administering sugar to a patient in diabetic coma may not reverse the situation, neither will it do increased harm. Insulin should never be administered to a person who is in a state of insulin shock. A person in a state of insulin shock may appear to breathe in a more shallow pattern, as opposed to a person experiencing a diabetic coma, whose breathing may be more rapid, deep, and labored in nature.

Additionally, the clinical athletic trainer should be cognizant of the fact that sensational deficits often accompany the diabetic patient.[5] Knowing this raises the athletic trainer's awareness of caution when applying thermal agents such as hot packs to an injured area. The inability to recognize temperature changes may result in burns from an uncomfortable treatment or an insufficient amount of layers of protection. Any decrease in circulatory function may also hinder the ability to dissipate heat.

The inability to properly perceive pressure and temperature changes often may result in open wounds. These wounds have a tendency to produce an environment highly conducive to invasion of foreign bodies and heal at very slow rates. The clinical athletic trainer should take care when applying such devices as ankle weights tightly around the patient's extremities so as not to create skin breakdown. Likewise, removal of any adherent pads or dressings should be done very carefully. Of course, therapeutic modalities should be used with caution and based upon the level of sensation with which a person presents.

NERVOUS SYSTEM

Epilepsy

Epilepsy can be defined as the temporary disturbance of the electrical impulses of the brain. This often results in involuntary convulsive movements, often called seizures. The treatment approach for dealing with seizures is no different in the traditional versus non-traditional setting. However, the circumstances surrounding the environment may present with a slightly different handling of the post-convulsion events when in a clinical setting.

The two forms of epilepsy that have been described are referred to as petit mal and grand mal.[6] A *petit mal* episode consists of a short duration, low level, twitching seizure that rarely involves the loss of consciousness. A *grand mal* episode is considered to be more dramatic in that violent, shaking convulsions may appear, a loss of consciousness occurs, and often a person will awake with appearances of foaming at the mouth and possibly a loss of bladder control. Upon awakening from a grand mal seizure, the person may feel extremely groggy and uncertain of the details to the particular circumstance.

Implications for Athletic Trainers

Prevention of seizures may only be controlled via the intervention of medication. Proper supervision in the clinical setting enables the ATC to communicate with a patient who suspects the onset of a seizure. A person may experience tinnitus and tingling in the fingers or toes, and may even complain of seeing "spots." These warning signs are called an "aura," and predictably signal the onset of a seizure. The ATC who is aware of an aura can adequately prepare for the episode to come. This would involve ensuring the safety of the individual as well as any other patients in the vicinity. Positioning the individual in a comfortable, level surface will reduce the risk of injury from falling. If possible, objects that may have the potential to cause harm should the individual come in contact with them should also be removed from the area.

Following the seizure, it is important for the clinical athletic trainer to maintain control of the environment. Human nature has determined that onlookers will be interested in the outcome. Although other observers may truly care and have the best intent of the individual in mind, it is important to ensure proper medical attention by trained staff and personnel only. It is also important to respect the dignity of the individual who has seized, especially if he or she has had an episode of a loss of bladder control. This can be quite embarrassing, and all attempts to reduce the embarrassment of the situation should be made.

Again, taking a thorough medical history helps the trainer to become more familiar with an individual's medical status. When an athletic trainer is made aware that a patient has a history of epilepsy, further inquisition should be made to determine the frequency and severity of the episodes, as well as the predisposing factors that precipitate the seizures, if known. Complete and accurate documentation is essential so that all members of the rehabilitation team are made aware of special concerns.

RESPIRATORY SYSTEM

As the nontraditional athletic trainer ventures into clinical, corporate, and industrial settings, he or she is more likely to treat a population of individuals that not only have orthopedic problems, but also underlying respiratory changes that may affect their overall performance in rehabilitation. The shift of importance to preventive medicine in today's world already has shown that a number of companies are encouraging their employees to take part in exercise programs. This has resulted in a larger number of physically active individuals requesting the services of athletic trainers. It has also resulted in more individuals, who previously did not take good care of their bodies, to begin seeking physiological changes. Regardless of the impetus for change, athletic trainers must be prepared to deal with those individuals who have less than optimal respiratory function as a result of detraining.

The primary function of the respiratory system is to provide for a transfer of air between the body and the environment. Many structures, including the pharynx, trachea, larynx, bronchi, bronchioles, alveoli, and lungs help to make up the complex respiratory system. In addition, the efficiency and flow of oxygen relies heavily on the muscles of inspiration, including the diaphragm and external intercostals. It should be noted that expiration is primarily an involuntary, passive movement.[7,8]

There are a number of respiratory conditions that an athletic trainer may stumble upon when working with the physically active person who is being treated for an orthopedic pathology. *Chronic obstructive pulmonary disease* (COPD) is a basic term used to describe a condition whereby the actual exchange of gases is ineffective.[10,11] These persons will exhibit a decreased vital capacity, and therefore will have a lower tolerance to exercise. *Dyspnea on exertion* (DOE) is common and would require the athletic trainer to implement frequent rests between exercise activities.

Included in the classification of COPD are chronic bronchitis, emphysema, and asthma. *Chronic bronchitis* is an inflammation of the bronchi. By definition, it is only chronic if it leads to an irritable and productive cough that lasts up to 3 months and occurs over at least 2 consecutive years.[12] This condition will usually be associated with heavy smokers. Athletic trainers may find themselves treating any number of respiratory conditions if a person has a history of smoking. Therefore, this should be determined when obtaining a medical history. Not only will frequent rests be indicated, but the initial implementation of an exercise program should start at less challenging levels, and must always be accompanied by a physician's approval for an exercise program.

Emphysema involves the destruction of the bronchioles and alveoli by nature of weakening and rupturing of the normally elastic structures. Factors contributing to emphysema are heavy cigarette smoking and air pollution. This respiratory condition is characterized by an abnormal posture demonstrating a forward head and rounded shoulders. In addition, a classic sign is the clubbing of fingers.[13] This condition presents with the same exercise concerns as does bronchitis. However, the individual with emphysema may also exhibit decreased mobility in the chest muscles and rib area as a result of poor posture and inflation of air into the lungs. This posture can be a predisposing factor to such orthopedic conditions as thoracic outlet syndrome, shoulder impingement, and cervical and thoracic strains.

Many athletic trainers are familiar with *asthma*, and recognize it as a condition that produces bronchospasms as a result of hypersensitivity to either the trachea, bronchi, or both. Although this is not inherited, it is believed that there may be a hereditary factor involved. However, diagnosis may be somewhat complicated.[14] With asthma, the process of expiration becomes difficult, and the person appears to be excessively and rapidly inspiring. Clinically, it is believed that episodes may be triggered by tense or emotional situations. Exposure to irritants in the air such as second-hand smoke or aerosol sprays may also trigger an asthmatic episode. Therefore, controlling the environment that one exercises in may help to prevent asthma attacks.

Implications for Athletic Trainers

Working with physically active patients who have underlying respiratory limitations can be a challenging and frustrating task for the athletic trainer. In order to improve a person's cardiorespiratory health status, he or she must exercise. However, extreme caution should be taken to avoid over-exerting an individual. First and foremost, an athletic trainer should have documented statements from a physician indicating that an individual is cleared to take part in a supervised exercise program. Specific questions or concerns should be clearly addressed prior to the initiation of any program.

Patients with *exercise induced asthma* (EIA) typically complain of shortness of breath, chest tightness, coughing, and/or wheezing 8–12 minutes following exercise of at least moderate intensity. This condition is a very common disorder affecting 3% to 7% of the adult population and is most prevalent in asthmatics.[15] In sports, where the difference between winning and losing can be measured in tenths of a second, this condition, if not diagnosed and properly treated, can have profound results. For the physically active industrial worker, this condition can dramatically reduce the work production during a given day if not correctly treated.

Athletic trainers are encouraged to work closely with the rehabilitation team when treating those who possess respiratory deficits. Members of the team in this case may include the physician, exercise physiologist, respiratory therapist, physical therapist, and nurse. Concentration should be focused on improving the status of the muscles of inspiration. This can be done directly through teaching proper mechanisms of breathing, or indirectly by improving the individual's posture. In addition, if the cause of the respiratory condition is known, such as smoking, education involving the importance of lifestyle change is essential. Rehabilitation of orthopedic conditions for the physically active person with respiratory deficiencies must not overlook the seriousness of that individual's endurance as it relates to exercise. For example, while an athletic trainer might normally use an upper body ergometer for rehabilitation of a shoulder injury, or a stationary cycle for the rehabilitation of a knee injury, a thorough assessment and consultation should indicate the level of resistance and the length of time for which a respiratory deficient patient should exercise.

Prevention is also a key. Avoidance of cold, dry air seems to play a role in preventing asthma attacks. Exercising in warmer environments, or even covering one's face with a mask or material that would facilitate warmth during exercise is recommended. Exercise in a pool appears to have clinical benefits because the environment is conducive to the asthmatic patient. Although increasing the physical endurance level for a person can also help to prevent the prevalence of attacks, caution should be taken by that person to avoid strenuous exercise during or soon after a respiratory infection.

Table 18-1
Risk Factors for Coronary Heart Disease

Age	Poor diet	Electrocardiographic abnormalities during rest and exercise
Gender	Hereditary components	
Elevated blood lipids	Personality and behavior patterns	
Hypertension		Family history
Cigarette smoking	High uric acid levels	Increased tension and stress levels
Physical inactivity	Pulmonary function abnormalities	
Obesity		
Diabetes mellitus	Race	

CARDIOVASCULAR SYSTEM

Hypertension

Hypertension implies blood pressure above normal limits and is possibly the most common chronic medical condition in the United States, affecting almost one-fourth of the population. It is often referred to as being either primary or secondary. *Primary hypertension* is the main condition and its etiology is relatively unknown. *Secondary hypertension* relates to high blood pressure that results from another underlying disease or condition.[16]

The danger of this common, often asymptomatic, readily detectable, and easily treatable condition lies in the end organ damage. Renal diseases, cerebral vascular accidents (CVA), and coronary artery diseases (CAD) may eventually evolve in untreated persons.[16,17] Therefore, it is imperative to be aware of the problem, its significance, and what impact it may have in the treatment plan of the active population. Newnan has outlined a list of the more frequently implicated risk factors that can be used to identify those at high or low risk for coronary heart disease (Table 18-1).[18]

The majority of cases of hypertension have no known etiology, but genetics and environment may play a role. A positive family history for hypertension significantly increases the chances of an individual developing hypertension. African Americans develop hypertension more often, at an earlier age, and at a more severe level than Caucasians. In a young patient population, hypertension is greater for males than females, but this reverses later in life. Hypertension has been shown to generally increase in both genders with respect to age. Overall morbidity and mortality increases progressively with higher levels of blood pressure. Other contributing factors intimately involved in the development and long-term risks of hypertension include obesity, cigarette abuse, dyslipidemia, diabetes mellitus, and physical inactivity.

As health care professionals, athletic trainers should be comfortable with taking a patient's blood pressure and are strongly encouraged to measure blood pressure as part of every patient's medical record. This additional health care monitoring of the patient can be extremely beneficial in the overall management of the hypertensive individual. Hypertension, however, should not be diagnosed on the basis of a single measurement. Initial elevated readings should be confirmed on at least two subsequent visits over a several week period, with average readings being greater than 140/90 required for diagnosis.[19]

Implications for Athletic Trainers

Athletic trainers can play a significant role in the treatment and management of hypertension by being familiar with the role of exercise in lowering blood pressure and the guidelines for exercise prescription and safety. There is now excellent data showing that regular aerobic exercise does lower blood pressure, although the exact mechanism is not completely understood.[20,21] The American College of Sports Medicine recommends 20–30 minutes of aerobic exercise three to four times per week at 70% of maximum heart rate for normotensives.[22]

However, the physical activity need not be complicated, and for most sedentary patients moderate activity such as brisk walking is beneficial. The majority of patients with mild hypertension can safely increase their level of physical activity without an extensive medical evaluation. Patients over the age of 45, however, must have a screening exercise treadmill test performed. Therefore, by documenting the blood pressure response to exercise, the patient can be instructed on the safest heart rate window for his or her exercise prescription.

Although aerobic exercise training is beneficial, patients with hypertension must be very careful with heavy resistance training. Potentially dangerous increases in blood pressure may be seen with heavy resistance or isometric training. By contrast, high repetition, low resistance weight training may effectively lower blood pressure without the potential adverse cardiovascular risks.[23]

Generally most physicians will try a 3- to 6-month trial of nonpharmacologic therapy including exercise in the management of hypertension. This approach may not be successful in controlling the blood pressure, at which time pharmacological therapy may be prescribed. These medicines are certainly important aspects of the treatment of hypertension, and the athletic trainer must be aware of the potential side effects of each class of drugs that may affect their safe use in a physically active population.

DISEASES OF THE BLOOD

Infectious Mononucleosis

Infectious mononucleosis is a very common, self-limiting lymphoproliferative disease caused by the Epstein-Barr Virus (EBV). It predominantly presents clinically in adolescent and young adults and is spread mainly by exchange of saliva. The incubation period is between 30 and 50 days. Infectious mononucleosis presents initially with a several day precursor of fatigue, headache, anorexia, and myalgia.[24]

The subsequent clinical picture consists of a 5- to 15-day history of fever, sore throat, and tender, enlarged cervical lymph nodes. Petechiae, a minute reddish or purplish spot containing blood, may be seen on the posterior palate of the throat. Palpable splenomegaly occurs in a good portion of the cases, along with occasional enlargement of the liver. The entire clinical course usually involves weeks rather than days.[25]

Diagnosis is made by history, physical exam, atypical lymphocytes on blood smear, and a positive serological slide test such as the mono spot. The mono spot and similar tests are accurate and sensitive, but it may take 2-3 weeks before the test reveals a positive result, and about 10% of adults will have a persistently negative test regardless.[25]

The most common cause of death from infectious mononucleosis is splenic rupture. Although rare, the risk certainly increases with the trauma of contact activity or performing activities like weight lifting that involve valsalva-like maneuvers. Most splenic ruptures occur during the first 2-3 weeks of the illness. If rupture does occur, the pain will begin abruptly in the left upper quadrant of the abdomen, and increases with inspiration. The pain may also be referred to the left shoulder (Kehr's sign). Computed tomography and ultrasound are the most frequently utilized diagnostic tests to confirm a splenic rupture. Surgery is usually required, but there is a growing trend towards nonsurgical observation and management, depending on the severity of the condition.

Implications for Athletic Trainers

No specific treatment exists for infectious mononucleosis, in which case supportive therapy usually suffices. Most patients feel much better in 2-3 weeks, but the highly trained individual and the poorly trained individual may both need extra time to regain functional levels of satisfaction.

The athletic trainer should be able to recognize the signs and symptoms of infectious mononucleosis because he or she may be the initial point of intervention for the patient. Symptoms such as fatigue, unexplained weight changes, and enlarged lymph nodes are not normal for any population, let alone the adolescent. Careful questioning and palpation of the abdominal quadrants can lead an athletic trainer to rule out or suspect splenic involvement as a relation to infectious mononucleosis. Identification of this condition should warrant a careful progression in rehabilitation regardless of the original cause of orthopedic injury. The patient should not return to contact activity until the spleen returns to normal size and is documented by appropriate testing. Additionally, blood studies should also return to pre-morbid levels. In most cases individual clinical judgment with cooperation of the physician is warranted to determine the most appropriate course of action.

Sickle Cell Disease

Sickle cell disease is a hemolytic hereditary disorder of primarily the African American population associated with a structural defect of the oxygen carrying hemoglobin molecules of the red blood cell. The abnormal hemoglobin results in a deformed red blood cell under states of reduced oxygen tension. This rigid spindle-shaped cell will not transverse easily through the blood vessels, therefore impairing oxygen delivery.[26]

In sickle cell disease an abnormal sickle cell gene is transmitted from each parent to the offspring. Most of the manufactured hemoglobin of the red blood cell is of the hemoglobin "S" type, resulting in a significant medical disorder associated with a severe hemolytic anemia, cardiovascular decompensation, and a painful organ infarction. Participation in sports is therefore usually very limited.

Sickle cell trait is usually a benign and asymptomatic condition in which the individual has one normal gene (Hemoglobin A) and one abnormal gene (Hemoglobin S), giving the genetic type "AS."[25] Sickle cell trait is seen in about 8% to 10% of the African American population in the United States, while sickle cell disease is present in less than 1%. The presence of sickle cell trait can be found in the physically active of all levels, and is not usually a barrier to outstanding performance.

Implications for Athletic Trainers

There are currently no accepted medical restrictions for the physically active with sickle cell trait. However, the National Collegiate Athletic Association (NCAA) Committee on

Competition Safeguards and Medical Aspects of Sports has determined the following points should be considered by athletic health care providers:

1. Routine sickle cell trait screening is not recommended.
2. No unwarranted restriction or limitation should be placed on an athlete with sickle cell trait.
3. All sickle cell trait athletes should be counseled to avoid dehydration; to acclimate gradually to heat, altitude, humidity, and exercise over time; and to refrain from extreme exercise during an acute febrile illness.[27]

The clinical athletic trainer should also take care to provide a safe environment, specifically one that prevents any patient from accidentally obtaining contusions, abrasions, or lacerations. Most importantly, with a sickle cell carrier, this person may be at greater risk to develop excessive bleeding following injury. This can very quickly become a medical emergency because this person already has been predisposed to impaired oxygen delivery to essential functioning tissue and organs.

Often the patient who has been diagnosed as having the sickle cell trait and/or disease will be well-versed with respect to the condition. An athletic trainer who is unfamiliar with the implications of the condition at hand should take time to educate him- or herself through conversations with the patient as well as through the utilization of additional reference materials.

Raynaud's Disease

Raynaud's disease is an arterial disorder in the form of a vasospasm, which subsequently decreases blood flow to the fingers and toes.[24,28] The decrease in blood flow results in sensory deficits, cyanosis, and pain to the localized areas. This condition is prevalent with exposure to cold or under stressful situations and is believed to have abnormalities of the sympathetic nervous system as its etiology.

Implications for Athletic Trainers

Although this condition is somewhat rare, it will inevitably cross the path of a clinical athletic trainer at one time or another. As with other nonorthopedic related medical disorders, a careful history that includes the appropriate questions can pick out a patient who does in fact have Raynaud's disease. Extreme measures should then be taken with the treatment of this individual when entertaining any thoughts of the application of ice or use of a cold whirlpool.

Treatment of an exacerbation can be accomplished by simple gradual warming of the involved area, at which time permanent deficits are rarely seen. However, the condition has been reported by patients to be quite painful, and so prevention is the key. Documentation of the condition should be made quite clear in a patient's chart of record so that any individual who is involved in the treatment of this patient will be able to clearly identify relevant precautions.

Hodgkin's Disease

Hodgkin's disease is a form of lymphoma in which a person's immune system becomes significantly impaired as the result of a virus that interferes with normal lymphocyte production.[24] This condition, which is fairly common in young athletes, initially presents with a painless enlargement in one lymph node, a fever, and an unexplained weight loss. Further progression of the condition may include the involvement of pathology to additional lymph tissues. Although classified as a malignant lymphoma, the actual malignant cells appear to remain in the lymph nodes as opposed to spreading throughout the circulatory system.

Implications for Athletic Trainers

The hallmark to Hodgkin's disease is the prevalence of long periods of remission that will follow an episode of illness. When first suspecting Hodgkin's as a possibility, the clinical athletic trainer should pay careful attention to the size and comparison of lymph nodes. Observation and palpation may reveal asymmetrical nodes, which can signify an early detection. In addition, patients have also described feelings of malaise and decreased interest with activity during the onset of this condition. Early intervention reveals good results, with many returning to their pre-morbid level of activity following adequate recovery time. However, the possibility of recurrence succeeding a long remission should not be forgotten.

INTEGUMENTARY SYSTEM

Athletic trainers are well versed with respect to dealing with many skin conditions that arise over the course of treating athletes and the physically active. However, one specific condition, psoriasis, needs to be discussed as it may present in any individual who is treated by an athletic trainer. This condition, like many other skin changes, has attached to it not only physical changes and characteristics, but also emotional implications.

Psoriasis

During the course of working with individuals who are physically active, an athletic trainer is sure to come in contact with a person who presents with a chronic type of skin disease known as psoriasis. Psoriasis is characterized by red patches of skin possessing sharply marked edges that are covered by scaly surfaces of skin. These scaly surfaces of skin have a high tendency to peel and shed from the body. This skin condition is said to be hereditary in nature, but it is not contagious.

This condition is characterized by periods of exacerbation and remission, and is believed to be aggravated by such conditions as stress, lack of sunlight, or any injury to the skin. Often lesions will present themselves around the extensor joint surfaces of the knees and elbows, yet in more severe cases they may spread throughout the entire body. The treatment for psoriasis may involve medications and other therapies such as ultraviolet radiation.

Implications for Athletic Trainers

Those persons being treated for an orthopedic condition who also present with a case of psoriasis will feel quite uncomfortable in the clinical setting where they may be on display for others to see. The athletic trainer would be doing this person a tremendous favor by using a private treatment room or a curtain that will enclose an otherwise open treatment area. Remember, the scaly surfaces of the skin will tend to fall off frequently, thus leaving a somewhat undesirable surface with which to work. It is important to be discrete in your attempts to work with this patient, as well as your attempts to cleanse and prepare the area for the next patient to be treated in that space. It is important again to respect the dignity of the individual and not to treat the person like he or she is different or inhumane. As a professional, the ATC owes it to this individual to instill a level of self-confidence and see through the superficial skin changes, as well as other orthopedic conditions, and treat this person as any other individual would be treated.

SUMMARY

The role of the athletic trainer is to return physically active people to their previous level of activity as quickly, but as safely, as possible. A common misconception exists among some that nonorthopedic problems do not impact athletic activity as significantly as orthopedic pathology. This is far from the truth. General medical problems not only impact the decision-making process in clearance for physical activity, but may have significant effects on the design of treatment and rehabilitation programs. Through the conduction of a detailed medical history and by having knowledge of pathophysiology and disease process, the athletic trainer can understand the relationship between the medical pathology and therapeutic treatment program, thus facilitating the highest quality of patient care.

Study Questions

1. Explain how the evolving clinical athletic trainer has become more responsible for recognizing nonorthopedic medical pathology.
2. What precautions would you as an athletic trainer take when working with a patient who knowingly has contracted HIV? How would you perform your duties while ensuring respect to the patient?
3. If you were working with a patient in the industrial setting who appeared to have signs of bulimia, how would you handle the situation? Would you confront the employee, or would you report your concerns to the employee's supervisor?
4. Assume that you are the athletic trainer assigned to work with a 54-year-old man who has undergone a total knee replacement 2 weeks ago. Past medical history reveals hypertension, diabetes mellitus, and previous carpal tunnel syndrome surgically treated 20 years ago. This person is complaining of severe pain that is accompanying moderate effusion. What treatment approach would you take with respect to addressing the symptoms of pain and effusion? Would you have any special concerns with any modalities or compression wraps?
5. When reviewing the medical chart for a 32-year-old woman whom you are treating for a mid-cervical strain, you identify that this woman has a history of seizures. What measures could you take to reduce the risk of seizures from occurring during your treatment sessions? If a seizure were to occur, what steps would you take to reduce the risk of injury to the patient?

6. While employed as an athletic trainer in an industrial setting, you notice that a fairly large number of employees whom you are treating for orthopedic conditions also have a history of respiratory illnesses. Is this a concern to you? How would you approach the employees about the health risks that this poses? Is this an issue that you feel is important enough to approach management? If so, how would you accomplish this?

7. When designing a cardiovascular rehabilitation program for an employee in an industrial setting who presents with a history of asthma, what special considerations would you implement in order to achieve optimal and safe results?

8. While taking a medical history from your patient, you inquire as to whether or not the patient is currently taking any medications. The patient responds by telling you that he takes one big blue pill and two yellow ones twice daily. How could you further determine the names of the medication that this person is taking? Following identification of the name of the medications, how would you go about determining the function of each? How would knowing the identity and function of these medications help you recognize additional pathology related to the person's current medical status?

9. How could you convince a patient with osteoarthritis of both knees that you are comfortable working with him or her regardless of the fact that there is an exacerbation of psoriasis and the patient feels very insecure?

References

1. 1993 Revised Classification System for HIV Infection. *CDC Morbidity and Mortality Weekly Report*.1992;41:1-3.

2. Hackman RM, Katra JE, Geersten SM. The athletic trainer's role in modifying nutritional behaviors of adolescent athletes: putting theory into practice. *J Ath Train*. 1992;27:262-267.

3. Chernoff R, Lipschitz DA. Nutrition and aging. In: Shils ME, Young VR, eds. *Modern Nutrition in Health and Disease*. 7th ed. Philadelphia, Pa: Lea & Febiger; 1988.

4. Mitchell CO, Chernoff R. Nutritional assessment of the elderly. In: Chernoff R, ed. *Geriatric Nutrition: The Health Professional's Handbook*. Gaithersburg, Md: Aspen Publishers; 1991.

5. Pfeifer MA, Greene DA. *Diabetic Neuropathy Current Concepts*. Kalamazoo, Mich: Upjohn; 1985.

6. American Academy of Orthopaedic Surgeons. *Athletic Training and Sports Medicine*. 2nd ed. Park Ridge, Ill; 1991.

7. Reid DC. Electromyographic studies of respiration: a review of current concepts. *Physiotherapy*. 1970;56:534-540.

8. Shaffer TH, Wolfson MR, Bhutani VK. Respiratory muscle function, assessment, and training. *Phys Ther*. 1981;61:1711-1723.

9. Soderberg GL. *Kinesiology: Application to Pathological Motion*. Baltimore, Md: Williams & Wilkins; 1986.

10. Petty T. Diagnosis and treatment of chronic obstructive pulmonary disease. *Chest*. 1990;97:1s-33s.

11. Carasso B. Therapeutic options in COPD. *Geriatrics*. 1982;37:99.

12. American Thoracic Society. Definitions and classification of chronic bronchitis, asthma, and pul-

monary emphysema. *American Review of Respiratory Diseases*. 1962;85:762.

13. Kisner C, Colby LA. *Therapeutic Exercise: Foundations and Techniques*. 3rd ed. Philadelphia, Pa: FA Davis; 1996.

14. Pratter MR, Hingston DM, Irwin RS. Diagnosis of bronchial asthma by clinical evaluation: an unreliable method. *Chest*. 1983;84:42.

15. Barnes P. *Asthma, in Bone: Pulmonary and Critical Care Medicine, Vol 1*. St. Louis, Mo: CV Mosby; 1993.

16. Sokolow M, McIlroy MB, Cheitlin MD. Clinical Cardiology. 5th ed. Norwalk, Conn: Appleton & Lange; 1990.

17. Goldberger E. *Essentials of Clinical Cardiology*. Philadelphia, Pa: JB Lippincott; 1990.

18. Newnan WB. Relation of serum lipoprotein levels and systolic blood pressure to early atherosclerosis: the Bogalusa study. *N Engl J Med*. 1986;314:138.

19. Mackler S. Instructional Lecture Notes. Newark, De: University of Delaware, Physical Therapy Program; 1993.

20. Blair SN, Painter P, Pate RR, Smith LK, Taylor CB. Resource Manual for Guidelines for Exercise Testing and Prescription. Philadelphia, Pa: Lea & Febiger; 1988.

21. Sannerstedt R. Hypertension. In: Skinner JS, ed. *Exercise Testing and Exercise Prescription for Special Cases: Theoretical Basis and Clinical Application*. Philadelphia, Pa: Lea & Febiger; 1987.

22. American College of Sports Medicine. *ACSM's Guidelines for Exercise Testing and Prescription*. 4th ed. Baltimore, Md: Williams & Wilkins; 1991.

23. Dean E, Ross J. Mobilization and Exercise Conditioning. In: Zadai C, ed. *Pulmonary Management in Physical Therapy*. New York, NY: Churchill Livingstone; 1992.

24. Carlton PJ, Mulvihill ML, Schanker NB. *Human Diseases: A Systematic Approach*. 4th ed. Norwalk, Conn: Appleton & Lange; 1995.

25. Kuland DN. *The Injured Athlete*. Philadelphia, Pa: JB Lippincott; 1988.

26. Bromberg PA, Ross DW. The Lungs and Hematologic Disease. In: Murray JF, Nadel J, eds. *Textbook of Respiratory Medicine*. Philadelphia, Pa: WB Saunders; 1988.

27. National Collegiate Athletic Association (NCAA) Committee on Competition Safeguards and Medical Aspects of Sports. Position Statement on Sickle Cell Anemia, Overland Park, Kansas; 1991.

28. Spittell JA. *Clinical Vascular Disease*. Philadelphia, Pa: FA Davis; 1983.

Suggested Readings

Afrasiabi R, Spector SL. Exercise induced asthma. *Phys Sport Med*. 1991;19:49-60.

American Academy of Pediatrics: Committee on Children with Handicaps and Committee on Sports Medicine. Sports and the Child with Epilepsy. *Pediatrics*. 1983;72:884-885.

American Association of Cardiovascular and Pulmonary Rehabilitation. *Guidelines for Cardiac Rehabilitation Programs*. 2nd ed. Champaign, Ill:Human Kinetics Publishers; 1991.

Anderson JC, Chopak JS, Bryant LD. Knowledge, attitudes, perception of risk, and preventive behaviors related to HIV/AIDS in college student athletes and nonathletes. *J Ath Train*. 1996;31:2(suppl);s-45. Abstract.

Clifton EJ, Clifton GD. Role of the athletic trainer in the use of inhaled bronchodilators. *J Ath Train*. 1989;24:325-328.

Cvengros RD, Lazor JA. Pneumothorax—a medical emergency. *J Ath Train*. 1996;31:167-168.

Dean E, Frownfelter D. *Principles and Practice of Cardiopulmonary Physical Therapy*. 3rd ed. St. Louis, Mo:CV Mosby; 1996.

Finnecy T, Mangus BC. Athletic participation after cardiac transplantation: a case study. *J Ath*

Train. 1989;24:224-226.

Foster DT, Rowedder LJ, Reese SK. Management of sorts-induced skin wounds. *J Ath Train*. 1995;30:135-142.

Gates JR. Epilepsy and sports participation. *Phy Sports Med*. 1991;19:98-104.

Harrelson GL, Fincher AL, Robinson JB. Acute Exertional Rhabdomyolysis and its relationship to sickle cell trait. *J Ath Train*. 1995;30:309-314.

Hodda JP, Badylak SF, May CL, Smith GF. Infective endocarditis in a collegiate wrestler. *J Ath Train*. 1995;30:105-108.

Irwin S, Tecklin JS. Cardiopulmonary Physical Therapy. St. Louis, Mo: CV Mosby; 1985.

Koberna T, Hoffman S. Pubic pain in a collegiate ice hockey player. *J Ath Train*. 1996;31:2(suppl);s-26. Abstract.

Leaver Dunn D, Robinson JB, KE Wright. Cardiopulmonary complaints in a high school football player. *J Ath Train*. 1996;31:2(suppl);s-26.

Lewis CB. *Aging: The Health Care Challenge*. 3rd ed. Philadelphia, Pa: FA Davis; 1996.

Lockette KF, Keyes AM. Conditioning with Physical Disabilities. Champaign, Ill: Human Kinetics Publishers; 1994.

Madaleno JA, Allen JR, Jacobson KE. Septic arthritis in a collegiate football player. *J Ath Train*. 1995;30:361-362.

Maddox J. Where the AIDS virus hides away. *Nature*. 1993;362:287.

Mueller MJ, Minor SD, Sahrmann SA, Schaff JA, Strube MA. Differences in the gait characteristics of patients with diabetes and peripheral neuropathy compared with age-matched controls. *Phys Ther*. 1994;74:299-308.

Noble HB, Porter M, Bach BR. Lyme disease in a young girl: case report. *Phys Sport Med*. 1989;17:135-141.

O'Sullivan SB, Schmidt TJ. Physical Rehabilitation: Assessment and Treatment. 3rd ed. Philadelphia, Pa: FA Davis; 1994.

Page P. Tourette syndrome in athletics: a case study and review. *J Ath Train*. 1990;25:254-259.

Pinger RR, Hahn DB, Sharp RL. The role of the athletic trainer in the detection and prevention of Lyme disease in athletes. *J Ath Train*. 1991;26:324-332.

Podolsky ML. Don't rule out sports for hypertensive children. *Phys Sports Med*. 1989;17:164-170.

Reid WD, Dechman G. Respiratory muscle testing for patients with chronic obstructive pulmonary disease. *Phys Ther*. 1995;75:996-1005.

Rothstein JM, Roy SH, Wolf SL. *The Rehabilitation Specialist's Handbook*. Philadelphia, Pa: FA Davis; 1991.

Sicard-Rosenbaum L, Lord D, Danoff JV, Thom AK, Eckhaus MA. Effects of continuous therapeutic ultrasound on growth and metastasis of subcutaneous murine tumors. *Phys Ther*. 1995;75:3-10.

Staten MA. Managing diabetes in older adults: how exercise can help. *Phys Sports Med*. 1991;19:3;66-77.

Whitely HL. HIV issues in athletics: Knowledge and attitude comparison between athletic directors and head trainers. *J Ath Train*. 1996;31:2(suppl);s-21.

Wiener CM. Exercise induced asthma. *J Ath Train*. 1989;24:6-11.

CHAPTER
19

Pharmacology

Robert S. Oziomek, MEd, ATC

OBJECTIVES

Upon completion of this chapter, the student will be able to accomplish the following:

1. Define pharmacology and explain its relationship to athletic training

2. Utilize correct drug nomenclature

3. Better understand the basic principles of pharmacology

4. List the various routes of administration of medications

5. Identify the different vehicles used to transport drugs into the body

6. Recognize different drugs used for the treatment of disorders of the nervous, cardiovascular, renal, respiratory, gastrointestinal, and endocrine systems

7. Identify common drugs used in the treatment of infectious diseases

Pharmacology, from the Greek words *pharmakon* (drug) and *logos* (a national discussion), is "the study of drugs; their sources, chemical and physical properties; physiologic actions; absorption; distribution; metabolism; excretion; and therapeutic uses."[1] In reality, a drug is any substance that has the ability to alter the structure or function of a living organism. Those drugs that possess useful properties are referred to as medicines.[2] Plants, minerals, and animals have all been used as drug sources due to their natural pharmaceutical or healing properties. Technology has allowed researchers to also manufacture drugs from artificial substances, creating what are known as synthetic drugs.

In the clinical setting it is likely that the athletic trainer will encounter some patients that are taking some form of medication. In some instances the patient may have been prescribed a drug to help treat the condition for which they are seeking therapy. However, in patient populations that cover a wide range of ages, the clinical athletic trainer is sure to find patients who are taking medications for other pre-existing conditions. As previously mentioned, a thorough medical history will reveal pertinent information with respect to medications. It is important to ask if the patient is currently taking any medications, including any over-the-counter (OTC) (nonprescription) drugs. After obtaining a list of medications, in many cases it will be necessary to ask the patient why the medication is being taken (i.e., what is the condition that the drug is treating). This may or may not be embarrassing to the patient, but in a professional manner the athletic trainer must assure the patient that this information is of great value, as it could affect the therapy treatment that the patient receives. In addition, the athletic trainer may not be aware of the purpose of a specific medication, and the patient's knowledge will therefore be of value. At no time should an athletic trainer implement a treatment without being fully aware of the condition, rationale, and side effects of a medication that a patient is taking. Questions directed to the patient should therefore address any side effects from the drug and whether or not the patient has been made aware by his or her doctor or pharmacist of any precautions that must be taken with the particular medication that has been prescribed. It has been suggested that rehabilitation can have an effect on a patient's response to certain medications, and in turn, that a patient's medication can determine the degree to which physical rehabilitation will be successful.[3-5] Ciccone has demonstrated this in his work to educate physical therapists.[3-5] Furthermore, treatment involving physical agents also may be influenced when administered to a client taking therapeutic drugs (Table 19-1).

This chapter will review the pharmacological actions that drugs produce in the body. Several classifications of drugs will be presented, and the impact that these medications and rehabilitation have on one another will be discussed.

DRUG LEGISLATION

Throughout the 20th century, the U.S. federal government adopted legislation to protect the consumer and control the drug market.[6,7] The Pure Food and Drug Act of 1906 required that all drugs be labeled accurately. This came from the concern that many medicine products contained addictive drugs. In 1938 the Food, Drug, and Cosmetic Act (Wheeler-Lea Act) called for proof from the manufacturers that a drug was safe before it was marketed. The Durham-Humphrey Amendment (1951) later established criteria for prescription and nonprescription drugs. Certain drugs were classified as "legend" drugs, and these drugs were to be prescribed by a physician. Testing procedures for new drugs were eventually established in 1962 with the Kefauver-Harris Amendment. Proof of a drug's safety and effectiveness was required in order for that drug to remain on the market. In 1970 the Comprehensive Drug Abuse Prevention and Control Act (Controlled Substances Act) created a category for drugs, such as depressants, stimulants, psychedelics, and narcotics, which had a high potential for abuse. The controlled substances were placed within one of five classifications, or "schedules," according to the potential for abuse:[8-11]

- **Schedule I**: High potential for abuse with limited or no medical use (e.g., heroin, LSD, marijuana).
- **Schedule II**: Restricted medical use with high potential for abuse that may lead to physical dependence (e.g., morphine, codeine, methadone, cocaine).
- **Schedule III**: Less potential for abuse than drugs listed in Schedule I and Schedule II, but use may result in limited dependence (e.g., anabolic steroids, methylpheridate, Tylenol with codeine).
- **Schedule IV**: Lower potential for abuse than Schedules I-III (e.g., phenobarbital, meprobamate, Valium, Librium).
- **Schedule V**: Potential for abuse is low (e.g., cough suppressants containing codeine and antidiarrheals containing paregoric, an opium tincture).

DRUG NOMENCLATURE

A drug can be identified by more than one name.[1,8,9,12] The chemical name describes the exact molecular formula of the drug. The generic name is assigned to the drug by the laboratory or company that first developed the drug. The generic name is often an abbreviation of the chemical name, and it is never capitalized. The manufacturer then gives its product a trade name or brand name. The trade name is copyrighted and used exclusively by that particular drug company.[9] The trade name is always capitalized and often appears in parentheses following the generic name. For example, ibuprofen (Advil®) and acetaminophen (Tylenol®) are common OTC pain relievers. The official name is the name by which the drug is referenced in The United States Pharmacopeia/National Formulary, and is usually the same as the generic name.[1,9]

In some cases a patient may not be familiar with medication(s) he or she has been prescribed. If this is the situation, it may be necessary for the clinical athletic trainer to obtain more information about a certain prescription drug with regard to any warnings, precautions, or side effects. An excellent resource is the *Physicians' Desk Reference* (PDR).[13] Advantages to using the PDR are that it is widely available, it is published annually, and it includes supplements throughout the year, keeping its information as up-to-date as possible.[5,9] The contents of the PDR are easily distinguished by its color-coded pages. The first section is the Manufacturers' Index (white pages) that lists all of the pharmaceutical companies contained in the PDR, including addresses and phone numbers. The Brand and Generic Name Index (pink pages) provides the reader with a page number of each product by brand name and generic name. The Product Category Index (blue pages) lists products by prescribing category (drug classification). The Product Identification Guide (gray pages) shows full-color, actual sized photos of tablets and capsules, arranged

Table 19-1

Potential Interactions Between Physical Agents and Therapeutic Drugs

Modality	Desired Therapeutic Effect	Drugs with Complementary/ Synergistic Effects	Drugs with Antagonistic Effects	Other Drug Modality Interactions
Cryotherapy Cold/ice packs Ice massage Cold baths Vapocoolant sprays	Decreased pain, edema, and inflammation	Anti-inflammatory steroids (glucocorticoids); nonsteroidal anti-inflammatory analgesics (aspirin and similar NSAIDS)	Peripheral vasodilators may exacerbate acute local edema	Some forms of cryotherapy may produce local vasoconstriction that temporarily impedes diffusion of drugs to the site of inflammation
	Muscle relaxation and decreased spasticity	Skeletal muscle relaxants	Nonselective cholinergic agonists may stimulate the neuromuscular junction	
Superficial and deep heat Local application Hot packs Paraffin Infrared	Decreased muscle/joint pain and stiffness Decreased muscle spasms	NSAIDs, opioid analgesics, local anesthetics Skeletal muscle relaxants	Nonselective cholinergic agonists may stimulate the neuromuscular junction	
Fluidotherapy Diathermy Ultrasound	Increased blood flow to improve tissue healing	Peripheral vasodilators	Systemic vasoconstrictors (e.g., alpha-1 agonists) may decrease perfusion of peripheral tissues	

continued

Table 19-1 (continued)

Potential Interactions Between Physical Agents and Therapeutic Drugs

Modality	Desired Therapeutic Effect	Drugs with Complementary/ Synergistic Effects	Drugs with Antagonistic Effects	Other Drug Modality Interactions
Systemic heat Large whirlpool Hubbard tank	Decreased muscle/joint stiffness in large areas of the body	Opioid and nonopioid analgesics, skeletal muscle relaxants		Severe hypotension may occur if systemic hot whirlpool is administered to patients taking peripheral vasodilators and some antihypertensive drugs (e.g., alpha-1 antagonists, nitrates, direct-acting vasodilators, calcium channel blockers)
Ultraviolet radiation	Increased wound healing	Various systemic and topical antibiotics		Antibacterial drugs generally increase cutaneous sensitivity to ultraviolet light (i.e., photosensitivity)
	Management of skin disorders (e.g., acne, rashes)	Systemic and topical antibiotics and anti-inflammatory steroids (glucocorticoids)	Many drugs may cause hypersensitivity reactions that result in skin rashes, itching	
Transcutaneous electrical nerve stimulation (TENS)	Decreased pain	Opioid and nonopioid analgesics	Opioid antagonists (naloxone)	
Functional neuromuscular electrical stimulation	Increased skeletal muscle strength and endurance		Skeletal muscle relaxants	
	Decreased spasticity and muscle spasms	Skeletal muscle relaxants	Nonselective cholinergic agonists may stimulate the neuromuscular junction	

Reprinted with permission from Ciccone CD. *Pharmacology in Rehabilitation.* 2nd ed. Philadelphia, Pa: FA Davis; 1996:600-602.

alphabetically by manufacturer. The main section of the PDR is the Product Information (also white pages). This section gives information on nearly 3,000 medications, including drug indications, effects, dosages, routes, methods and frequency, and duration of administration, as well as any relevant warnings, hazards, contraindications, side effects, or precautions. The drugs in this section are alphabetized according to manufacturer. The last section, Diagnostic Product Information (green pages), provides guidelines for use of common diagnostic agents. For OTC, the *Physicians' Desk Reference for Nonprescription Drugs* is also available as a resource.[14]

BASIC PRINCIPLES OF PHARMACOLOGY

The science of pharmacology can further be divided into the areas of *pharmacokinetics* and *pharmacodynamics*. Pharmacokinetics is the study of the absorption, distribution, biotransformation (metabolism), and excretion of a drug in the body.[5,15-17] Pharmacodynamics is the study of a drug's physiological effects and mechanisms of action.[5,12,15,16] Basically pharmacokinetics looks at "what the body does to the drug" and pharmacodynamics looks at "what the drug does to the body."[15]

Pharmacokinetics

Pharmacokinetics begins with absorption of the drug. Absorption occurs when the drug enters the bloodstream.[2,9,12] The rate and extent of absorption depends on several factors, including the solubility of the drug and the route of administration.[2,9,18] Distribution of a drug refers to its movement from the bloodstream into the tissues. Drug metabolism, or biotransformation, usually occurs in the liver, as the drug is chemically broken down. This process is the body's attempt to eliminate the drug.[12] A drug that is absorbed from the stomach and intestines goes directly to the liver where an initial breakdown takes place, before the active drug reaches the systemic circulation. This route through the liver is known as the "first-pass" effect.[12,18] The amount of the active drug that reaches the general circulation and can be distributed to its site of action is referred to as the drug's bioavailability.[18] Excretion is the elimination of the waste products from drug metabolism and usually occurs via the renal system.[2,9,12]

Pharmacodynamics

Pharmacodynamics explores the action of drugs on the body. The effectiveness of a drug is determined by its ability to alter the function of cells. All drugs create both cellular changes and physiological changes.[9] The cellular changes occur when the drug attaches itself to the specific receptor site of certain cells.[12] These cellular changes are referred to as the drug action.[9,12] The drug effect occurs as a result of the physiological changes that take place following the cellular changes. These drug effects can take place either systemically or locally.[9] However, no drug has only one effect on the body.[12] Other than its intended therapeutic effects, drugs also create side effects. Although these side effects are not desirable, they are generally not harmful.[12]

ROUTES OF ADMINISTRATION

One of the key factors in determining the effectiveness of a drug is its route of administration. There are several ways in which drugs can be introduced into the body. The choice of route is determined by the desired effects of the drug, absorption qualities of the drug, and how the drug is supplied.[9]

Enteral Routes

Enteral routes utilize the alimentary canal and include oral, sublingual, buccal, and rectal methods of administration. The *oral route* is most common, as it is easy, safe, and economical.[12,18] Medications taken by mouth (or PO) are swallowed, then absorbed from the gastrointestinal (GI) tract. In order for the drug to pass through the gastrointestinal mucosa into the bloodstream, it must have a (relatively high) degree of lipid solubility.[5] Once the drug is absorbed into the bloodstream, it is directly transported via the portal vein to the liver, where the drug in part will be metabolized and destroyed before ever reaching its site of action. This too is known as the first-pass effect.[5] The onset of action of drugs administered orally is approximately 30–60 minutes.[12] A disadvantage of the oral route is that some drugs can cause gastric irritation, and other medications are destroyed by stomach acids and digestive juices.[2,15]

The *sublingual route* of administration involves placing medication under the tongue. The drug is absorbed through the oral mucosa into the venous system. The drug will eventually be transported to the heart after it passes through the superior vena cava. Hence, a drug can reach the systemic circulation and avoid the first-pass effect of the liver if it is administered sublingually.[5,18] Nitroglycerin, used to treat angina pectoris, is administered in this fashion, and would otherwise be destroyed in the liver if it were to be absorbed from the stomach and intestines.[5] The sublingual route is used when rapid effects are needed and the onset of action is within several minutes.[12] Medication in the form of troches, or lozenges, can also be placed in the pouch of the cheek, that is by *buccal administration*, where the lozenge is slowly dissolved and the medication is absorbed by the mucous lining of the mouth.[19] *Rectal administration* of a drug is not as common due to the difficulty in regulating the dosage of the medication, but rectal suppositories can still be used to treat local conditions.[5,12]

Parenteral Routes

Parenteral routes of administration are methods that do not use the alimentary canal and include injections, topical application, transdermal application, and inhalation. These routes are utilized when the patient is unable to take medications PO, or the drug is not suitable for GI absorption.

Hypodermic injections can be subcutaneous, intramuscular, intravenous, intraarterial, or intrathecal.[5,12] *Subcutaneous injections* yield a local response, such as in the use of local anesthetics. Subcutaneous injections also allow for a slower release of the medication into the bloodstream.[5] This is desirable for insulin-dependent diabetics, as a slow release of insulin into the bloodstream helps to better control blood sugar levels. *Intramuscular (IM) injections* are used to treat specifically injured muscles, or as a means to release a drug into the bloodstream in a steady manner.[5] Common sites for IM injections include the gluteal muscle and the deltoid muscle.[19] IM injections are utilized when high blood levels of the drug are required and when rapid effects are desired, as the onset of action is within several minutes.[12] *Intravenous (IV) injections* allow for medications to be directly introduced into the bloodstream.[5] IV injections are used in emergency situations in which the immediate effects of a drug are required, as the onset of action is within 1 minute.[12] *Intraarterial injections* are rare and usually are limited to cancer drugs, when a local effect is desired on a specific organ.[5,12] *Intrathecal injections* are within the spinal subarachnoid space and are used for local effects (e.g., in spinal anesthetics).[5,12]

Topical medications are applied to the skin or mucous membranes. In the form of creams or ointments, topical medications are not readily absorbed into the bloodstream, and instead are used to treat local conditions on the skin.[5,12] *Transdermal medications* are delivered using medicated patches. Transdermal administration allows for a slow release of the drug into the bloodstream, thus maintaining relatively constant plasma levels of the drug over a period of time.[5] Common drugs that are introduced into the body transdermally include nitroglycerin and nicotine.[5] Iontophoresis and phonophoresis, common treatments utilized by clinical athletic trainers in treating musculoskeletal disorders, are also considered transdermal techniques.[5] Administration of a drug by inhalation is for local effects within the respiratory tracts, but it is difficult to determine how much of the drug actually reaches the target tissue.

DRUG VEHICLES

A substance that transports a drug into the body is known as a drug vehicle. Very often the dosage form is one of the key factors in determining the therapeutic effectiveness of a drug. Some of the more common pharmaceutical preparations are listed in Table 19-2.[1,9,19]

DRUG CLASSIFICATIONS

This section will present drug classifications with respect to their effect on particular systems within the body, as outlined by Hitner and Nagle.[12]

Pharmacology of the Peripheral Nervous System

The peripheral nervous system is comprised of 12 pairs of cranial nerves and 31 pairs of spinal nerves. This system can be divided into a somatic division and a visceral division. The *somatic nerves* are those nerves that branch from the cranial and spinal motor nerves to innervate skeletal muscle and are under voluntary control. The *visceral nerves* branch from the cranial and spinal motor nerves where they innervate cardiac and smooth muscle, and are not under conscious control (involuntary). These visceral nerves make up what is commonly known as the autonomic nervous system.

The autonomic nervous system can be further divided into the sympathetic division and parasympathetic division. The *sympathetic nerves* are stimulated during the "fight or flight" response, whereas the purpose of the *parasympathetic nerves* is to regulate body functions not requiring a great deal of energy expenditure.[12] From a pharmacological standpoint, the difference between sympathetic nerves and parasympathetic nerves lies in the neuro-

Table 19-2
Common Pharmaceutical Preparations

Oral Drug Forms

Capsule: drug contained within a gelatin receptacle

Lozenge (troche): a tablet containing a flavorable taste, used to treat local conditions in the mouth and throat

Elixir: liquid solution containing alcohol, sugar, and water

Emulsion: liquid drug form that contains oils and fats in water

Pill or tablet: powdered forms of a drug compressed into a suitable mold, such as a small oval or circle

Solution: liquid preparation in which the drug is completely dissolved in solution

Suspension: a liquid form of medication that requires shaking before use, as the drug is not evenly dissolved in the fluid medium

Syrup: liquid drug form that contains sugar as a sweetener

Rectal Drug Forms

Enema solution: drug in solution administered rectally as an enema

Suppository: mixture of a drug with a firm base substance, such as cocoa butter, that is inserted into a body orifice and melts at body temperature

Topical Drug Forms

Dermal patch: medicated skin patch that contains drug molecules that are absorbed through the skin at varying rates, allowing for a consistent level of the drug in the bloodstream

Liniment: a mixture of alcohol or oil with a dissolved drug, applied to the skin by rubbing or massage, to act as a counterirritant

Lotion: a liquid drug preparation that is used to treat skin conditions and is patted on, rather than rubbed on

Ointment or cream: a semisolid drug preparation that is applied externally, usually by rubbing

Injectable Drug Forms

Powder: dry drug particles are mixed with a sterile diluting solution, such as saline solution, prior to injection

Solution: drug suspended in a sterile water base (aqueous solution) or an oil base (viscous solution)

Inhalable Drug Forms

Gas: some general anesthetics are administered in a gaseous form utilizing the respiratory tract for administration

Powder: a special device called a spinhaler allows for a powdered drug, cromolyn sodium, to be inhaled for the relief of bronchial asthma

Spray or mist: liquid form of the drug that is inhaled as small droplets, using a nebulizer, spray bottle, or inhaler

transmitter that is released from the postganglionic nerve ending. The neurotransmitter at the postganglionic nerve endings in the parasympathetic nervous system is acetylcholine, but the neurotransmitter at the postganglionic nerve endings in the sympathetic nervous system is norepinephrine. Nerves that release acetylcholine are described as cholinergic, and nerves that release norepinephrine are described as adrenergic.[12]

Drugs that affect the sympathetic nervous system include the adrenergics and adrenergic blockers. Adrenergic drugs mimic the "fight or flight" of the sympathetic nervous system, resulting in cardiac stimulation, increased blood flow to skeletal muscles, and bronchodilation. These drugs are used to restore heart rhythm following a cardiac arrest and to increase blood pressure in shock of all kinds. Adrenergic blockers, or beta blockers, block the action of the sympathetic nervous system. Medications such as propranolol (Inderal®) are used to treat hypertension, angina pectoris, and cardiac arrythmia by decreasing heart rate and cardiac output.[9,12] The clinical athletic trainer should be aware that patients taking beta blockers should be slow to rise from a reclined position so as to avoid postural hypotension.[9]

Drugs that affect the parasympathetic nervous system include the cholinergics and the anticholinergics. Cholinergic drugs are used to prevent constipation and urinary retention after general anesthesia by stimulating GI and gerito-urinary peristalsis. These drugs are also used to treat glaucoma. Anticholinergic agents such as atropine are used to increase heart rate. Synthetic forms of the anticholinergic drugs have been used to treat GI disorders such as ulcers.[12]

Skeletal muscle relaxants inhibit skeletal muscle contraction. The clinical athletic trainer will find these medications useful in the rehabilitation of conditions that present with a decrease in range of motion due to muscle spasm. Dantrolene (Dantrium®) has a direct effect on skeletal muscles and is used to manage spasticity in conditions such as multiple sclerosis and cerebral palsy. Potential side effects include drowsiness, dizziness, weakness, and blurred vision. These side effects certainly could affect the outcome of a clinical treatment, so treatments should be conducted when sedative effects are at a minimum. Drugs such as chlordiazepoxide (Librium®) and diazepam (Valium®) are centrally acting muscle relaxants, but are mainly used as antianxiety drugs.

Local anesthetics are utilized to relieve pain without depressing the central nervous system the way general anesthetics do. When local anesthetics are used, there is a temporary loss of sensation or feeling in a targeted area without a decrease in alertness or mental function. It is possible that the athletic trainer may apply local anesthetics transdermally when using in intophoresis or phonophoresis as part of the treatment regimen. If a physician injects the patient with a local anesthetic, it would be wise to schedule treatments immediately following injections to facilitate exercise. Caution must be used, however, when choosing modalities, as sensation will be decreased.

Pharmacology of the Central Nervous System

The central nervous system (CNS) is made up of the brain and spinal cord. The CNS acts to coordinate and control the activity of the body's other systems. The way in which medications act on the CNS is by affecting neurotransmitters.

Drugs that are utilized to depress the CNS are referred to as sedative-hypnotic medications. These drugs combat the anxiety, worry, tension, and fear that accompanies mental stress. The sedative-hypnotic drugs can be divided into two major types: the barbiturates and the nonbarbiturates. In small dosages, the sedative-hypnotics promote sedation, and in larger doses they promote sleep. It is advised not to schedule patients for treatments shortly after these drugs have been administered if they produce significant sedation, especially if a great deal of patient participation is required for the treatment. The barbiturate drug phenobarbital is also used in the treatment of seizure disorders.

Tranquilizers are drugs that are used to create calmness and peace of mind in patients with mental illness, but without producing sedation or mental confusion. These medications can be divided into antipsychotic drugs (major tranquilizers) and antianxiety drugs (minor tranquilizers). The antipsychotic drugs appear to have a selective effect on the thalamus and limbic system, which regulate behavior. Many of these drugs fall into the category of phenothiazines and are used to treat the symptoms of psychoses or severe neuroses, including delusions and hallucinations. Because these drugs normalize patient behavior, therapy should be enhanced in patients who have been prescribed antipsychotic drugs. Although less serious effects of these drugs such as sedation and orthostatic hypotension might be present, a much more serious problem is extrapyramidal motor effects. Any change in posture, balance, or involuntary motor movements should be reported to the physician so that appropriate alterations in medication and/or dosage can be made in order to avoid long-term or permanent motor dysfunction.[5] The antianxiety drugs act mainly on the limbic system and spinal cord and are used to calm the patient and reduce the symptoms of anxiety. These drugs are used in the short-term treatment of anxiety disorders. Although meprobamate was one of the first antianxiety drugs to be used, diazepam (Valium) and chlordiazepoxide (Librium) are more common today.[9,12] Because these drugs create a calming effect in the patient, it is wise to schedule treatments when the drugs are at peak levels to ensure the patient's cooperation, assuming sedation does not occur.

Central nervous system stimulants act to promote CNS function. The drug methylphenidate (Ritalin®) is used in the treatment of attention deficit disorder (ADD) in children over the age of 6 years and is also used in cases of narcolepsy.[9] There can be some side effects in patients on this medication, including irritability, headache, blurred vision, nausea, and vomiting. Athletic trainers dealing one-on-one with patients on Ritalin may be able to provide valuable input in determining the effectiveness of the drug.

Patients suffering from depression often experience changes in mood and behavior, accompanied by feelings of frustration and hopelessness. There are several types of antidepressants, or "mood elevators," to treat this condition. Two broad categories of the drugs include the tricyclics and the monoamine oxidase (MAO) inhibitors. Also, another common drug to treat depression is fluoxetine (Prozac®). Side effects of Prozac include nausea, anxiety, nervousness, and insomnia. Lithium is another drug used in the long-term treatment of major depression and bipolar disorders (manic depressive disorders). Although patients may be on antidepressants to improve their overall mood, these drugs can also be prescribed to patients suffering from a spinal cord injury, stroke, severe burn, multiple sclerosis, or amputation. The antidepressants may help the patient become more optimistic about the outcome of the treatment plan, and this is likely to make the patient more cooperative throughout the rehabilitation process. Sedation and muscle weakness can occur with the use of the tricyclics and lithium, however, and orthostatic hypotension is another side effect that occurs with the tricyclics. Therefore caution should be taken when a patient is asked to perform an exercise that will elevate blood pressure.

Epilepsy is a medical condition that is characterized by periodic seizures, which are a result of abnormal electrical activity in the brain, especially in the cerebral cortex. These seizures may result in a momentary loss of consciousness and an episode of involuntary muscle twitching or convulsions. Antiepileptic drugs act to reduce the number and/or severity of seizures in patients with epilepsy by decreasing nerve excitability. The athletic trainer should always be made aware of any patient who has had a history of seizures and is presently taking medication to control seizures in order to recognize and deal with the onset of a seizure. Side effects of antiepileptic drugs such as headache, dizziness, sedation, nausea, and vomiting may hinder rehabilitation treatments. Skin conditions, such as dermatitis or a rash, can occur with the long-term use of antiepileptic drugs. The athletic trainer should avoid any therapeutic modalities that could worsen these skin conditions. In some epileptics, their seizures tend to be set off by environmental stimuli such as sound or light. Other seizures tend to be triggered at certain times during the day. With those points in mind, it is recommended that epileptic patients be scheduled during a time when the clinical setting is relatively quiet and there is a low risk of a seizure.

Skeletal muscle tone and body movement is regulated in part by the basal ganglia within the medulla of the cerebrum. Parkinson's disease is a condition in which damage has occurred to the basal ganglia, resulting in muscle tremors, rigidity, muscle weakness, shuffling gait, and other disturbances in movement and postural balance.[9,12] Parkinson's disease can be caused by infections, brain tumors, arteriosclerosis, and excessive administration of certain types of drugs (antipsychotic drugs). There are different classes of drugs used to treat Parkinson's disease. Generally these drugs are all referred to as anti-Parkinson drugs because they all act on the neurotransmitters that affect the basal ganglia. Larodopa (L-dopa®) is one of the more common anti-Parkinson drugs. Most of the anti-Parkinson drugs cause orthostatic hypotension, so the athletic trainer must be extremely careful in dealing with patients who have Parkinson's disease because the rehabilitation program for these patients includes gait training and balance exercises. It has been suggested that patients taking anti-Parkinson drugs be scheduled approximately 1 hour after ingesting their medication so that the peak effects of the drug help benefit the treatment session.

General anesthetics act to depress the central nervous system and are typically used during surgery to prevent the reaction to painful stimuli. Under anesthesia, a patient loses all sensations, because hearing, sight, touch, and pain are all absent.[12] Athletic trainers who deal with patients the same day as their surgery or even the day after their surgery may encounter patients who have not fully recovered from the effects of the anesthesia.[5] General anesthetics tend to make the patient woozy, and certain types of anesthetics can produce confusion and psychotic behavior as the patient recovers. The athletic trainer should incorporate appropriate treatment activities during this recovery time, as muscle weakness can also occur as a result of the anesthesia.

Narcotic analgesics are drugs that are capable of inhibiting painful stimuli and are used primarily to relieve severe pain of trauma and terminal illness, and also to relieve postoperative pain.[5,12] The narcotics are derived from opium or synthetic chemicals similar to opium. Examples of natural narcotic analgesics include morphine and codeine. Tolerance and physical dependence can occur with chronic use of narcotics. Patients taking narcotic analgesics may experience sedation and GI discomfort, but the pain relief associated with the drug will likely benefit the rehabilitation program. Hence, patients on narcotic analgesics should be scheduled for treatments when the drug is at a peak level in their systems. The athletic trainer should be aware that narcotics can cause respiratory depression, and thus exercise intensity should be monitored very carefully when patients have been prescribed this medication.[5,9]

Nonnarcotic analgesics are also used to treat pain, but are more effective for the low to moderate intensity pain associated with dull aches and inflammation. Although the nonnarcotic analgesics are not effective against severe pain, they do not contain any opium-like substances, and therefore do not produce tolerance or physical dependence. Nonnarcotic analgesics act on the CNS like the narcotic analgesics do to decrease pain, but the nonnarcotic analgesics differ in that they also produce a peripheral mechanism of action. A common group of nonnarcotic analgesics is the salicylates. Acetylsalicylic acid (aspirin) is widely used not only for its analgesic effect, but also for its antipyretic effect, antiinflammatory effect, and anticoagulant effect. However, aspirin can irritate the stomach lining, and for that reason, other medications are chosen over aspirin. Acetaminophen (Tylenol) is a relatively safe alternative to aspirin. Often included in the category of nonnarcotic analgesics are the antiinflammatory drugs more commonly known as nonsteroidal antiinflammatory drugs (NSAIDS). These drugs inhibit the synthesis of prostaglandins, which are responsible for producing pain and inflammation. NSAIDS such as ibuprofen (Motrin®) and naproxen (Naprosyn®) are commonly used to treat orthopedic conditions. NSAIDS may cause stomach upset, so it is usually recommended that these medications be ingested with food. There are no other significant side effects of NSAIDS, which makes them a valuable supplement to the rehabilitation program, as they provide pain relief, which can facilitate exercise.

Pharmacology of the Heart

Cardiac glycosides are prescribed to patients suffering from congestive heart failure (CHF) to strengthen the heartbeat. These drugs act on the myocardium to increase the force of contraction, therefore increasing cardiac output. The cardiac glycosides are derived from the plant leaves of Digitalis purpurea and Digitalis lanata. Common cardiac glycosides include digoxin (Lanoxin®) and digitoxin (Crystodigin®). Side effects of the cardiac glycosides include headache, fatigue, muscle weakness, and vertigo. During treatment sessions, athletic trainers should recognize signs of acute congestive heart failure, such as increased dyspnea, rales, cough, and frothy sputum. Patients with CHF may be taking other medications, also, including vasodilators and diuretics. Those drugs will be discussed in a later section.

Cardiac arrhythmias are disturbances in normal cardiac rhythm and are not uncommon. Arrhythmias may be a result of a diseased heart or a result of chronic drug therapy. Antiarrhythmic drugs do not cure arrhythmias, but instead restore the normal cardiac rhythm. These drugs suppress various types of arrhythmias, such as atrial or ventricular tacchycardia and atrial fibrillation, by lowering blood pressure and heart rate. Adrenergic blockers, such as propranolol (Inderal), correct the arrhythmias by inhibiting adrenergic (sympathetic) nerve receptors. Calcium blockers, such as verapamil, diminish the action of calcium in the contraction of the heart muscle, and therefore reduce its excitability. Other antiarrhythmia agents include lidocaine and quinidine. A serious side effect with antiarrhythmic drugs is the possibility of increased arrythmia or changes in the nature of arrhythmias, especially with patients who are exercising. Electrocardiogram (ECG) recordings monitored by a knowledgeable clinician would detect such arrhythmias, but that clinical set-up is not always available. However, checking the patient's pulse for rate and regularity to possibly detect rhythm disturbances, and also being aware of other symptoms such as faintness and dizziness, may lead the athletic trainer to suspect occurring arrhythmias. Other side effects are minor. Some antiarrhythmic drugs may cause hypotension, and dizziness may occur if the patient abruptly changes posture.

Antianginal agents, or coronary vasodilators, are used to treat angina pectoris. Angina pectoris is characterized by periodic episodes of severe chest pain due to decreased blood flow to the heart. This decreased blood flow is usually due to a thickening of the coronary arteries. The antianginal drugs act by relaxing vascular smooth muscle, which produces arterial vasodilation, thus lowering blood pressure and decreasing venous return to the heart. Hence less oxygen is required by the heart and chest pain is relieved. Coronary vasodilators used to manage angina prophylactically include beta blockers, calcium blockers, and nitrates. One of the more common nitrates is nitroglycerin. Nitroglycerin can be administered in sublingual tablets. If the angina is not relieved after one tablet, additional nitroglycerin tablets can be taken every 5 minutes, not to exceed three total tablets in a 15-minute period. If pain still persists after three dosages, this could indicate an acute myocardial infarction, and a physician should be contacted immediately. Nitroglycerin can also be administered transdermally, with nitroglycerin patches applied to the upper arm or body, and not below the elbow or knee. These patches are usually changed every 24 hours, and sites should be rotated so as to avoid skin irritation. Patients who take nitroglycerin only at the onset of an acute angina episode should always have their medication available during treatment sessions because exercise performed during rehabilitation can increase the heart's demand for oxygen. It is not as critical for patients taking nitroglycerin prophylactically to have their medication with them during rehabilitation, but the athletic trainer must recognize the limitations of these patients when prescribing exercise. Some antianginal drugs increase a patient's tolerance to exercise, while others decrease the patient's ability to handle higher exercise workloads. Hypotension as a result of peripheral vasodilation can be a side effect of the nitrates and calcium blockers. Warm whirlpool submersion and even exercise alone can create an additional peripheral vasodilation response, which could result in dizziness and syncope. For this reason, modalities should be carefully chosen.

Pharmacology of the Vascular and Renal Systems

Diuretics are drugs that act to increase urinary excretion. The thiazide drugs are the most frequently used diuretics, and are prescribed for the treatment of edema, hypertension, and electrolyte imbalance resulting from renal dysfunction. The nonthiazide drugs, such as furosemide (Lasix®) and bumetanide (Bumex®), act more rapidly and are more effective than the thiazide drugs. The nonthiazide drugs are used to treat CHF, edema due to renal failure, hypertension, and pulmonary edema. Patients who are prescribed diuretics can possibly develop fluid and electrolyte depletion.

Vigorous exercise and warm whirlpool submersion could potentially contribute to this problem. The athletic trainer may be able to detect early warning signs, such as excessive fatigue and weakness. Patients taking diuretics should be instructed to rise slowly from a seated or reclined position. Also be aware that treatment sessions may be interrupted by the patient's need to use the restroom facilities.

Hypertension is simply defined as abnormally high blood pressure in the arterial system. This condition is one of the leading causes of cerebral strokes, heart attacks, and kidney disease.[12] Two factors which generally determine blood pressure are cardiac output and peripheral resistance. Peripheral resistance is increased during vasoconstriction. Antihypertensive drugs have various modes of action, but all work to lower blood pressure.

Rauwolfia alkaloids, beta adrenergic blockers (e.g., propranolol [Inderal]) and calcium blockers (e.g., diltiazem [Cardizem®]) are all classified as antihypertensives.[9] Various diuretics and vasodilators can also be used to treat hypertension. Because most of the antihypertensives act by lowering blood pressure, it is not uncommon for patients on these medications to experience hypotension and orthostatic hypotension. Hence, posture changes should be executed carefully. When vasodilating drugs are used to control hypertension, activities that cause further vasodilation, such as warm whirlpool submersion and exercise, must be monitored carefully, if not avoided altogether. If beta blockers are used, the patient's tolerance to exercise will be somewhat diminished.

Anticoagulants are drugs that prevent blood clots from forming or decrease the extension of existing blood clots in conditions such as venous thrombosis, pulmonary embolism, and coronary occlusion. Anticoagulants fall into two general categories: heparin and the coumadin derivatives. Heparin is always administered either intravenously or subcutaneously, as this drug is not absorbed from the GI tract. The coumadin derivatives (e.g., Coumadin) interfere with the action of vitamin K in order to disrupt the coagulation process. These drugs are given by mouth and are used more commonly for long-term anticoagulation therapy. Patients taking anticoagulant drugs should avoid all other medications (especially aspirin, antiinflammatory drugs, and antacids) unless approved by the patient's physician. Patients who take anticoagulants are at risk for increased bleeding; therefore, manual techniques (e.g., deep tissue massage) should be employed with caution so as to not traumatize underlying tissues. Of course, safety is always a concern in the clinical setting. Extra attention should be given to the hydrotherapy to ensure that a wet and slippery condition does not lead to a fall that could result in extreme or internal bleeding in a patient taking anticoagulation drugs.

Pharmacology that Affect the Respiratory System

Antihistamines are drugs that are used to relieve allergy symptoms caused by the chemical histamine. Antihistamines work by attaching to the histamine receptor sites in an effort to decrease the swelling and itching associated with the release of histamine. Antihistamine drugs such as diphenhydramine (Benadryl®) are used to treat allergy symptoms. Antihistamines can cause drowsiness in some patients, so supervision is necessary for those patients when they are utilizing certain pieces of rehabilitation equipment. Decongestants such as pseudoephedrine (Sudafed®) are adrenergic in nature and work by constricting blood vessels in the respiratory tract, which decreases swollen mucous membranes and thus allows nasal passages to open.[9] OTC decongestants are often combined with other medications such as antihistamines and analgesics. Decongestants are administered orally and by nasal sprays, and should be used on a short-term basis only.

Bronchodilators increase the vital capacity of the lungs and relieve bronchospasm by relaxing the smooth muscles of the bronchial tree. Acute respiratory conditions such as asthma can be treated with bronchodilators, as can many forms of chronic obstructive pulmonary disease (COPD). The xanthine derivatives and the sympathomimetics (adrenergics) are two classifications of bronchodilators. Aminophyllin®, a theophylline drug, is a common xanthine derivative. Sympathomimetic drugs such as albuteral sulfate (Ventolin®, Proventil®) are available in aerosol form for inhalation in devices called metered dose inhalers. These inhalers are used commonly by athletes prior to competition to diminish exercise-induced asthma. Patients who utilize inhalers should be instructed to bring their medication with them to all treatment sessions, especially if the rehabilitation program includes exercise that could trigger bronchospasms.

Pharmacology of the GI Tract

During the digestive process, hydrochloric acid (HCI) and proteolytic enzymes such as pepsin are produced in the stomach to help break down food.[12] Antacids are OTC drugs that act to partially neutralize gastric HCI to relieve indigestion and heartburn. Antacids can also be prescribed to relieve pain and promote healing of gastric and duodenal ulcers. Most antacids contain aluminum, calcium carbonate, or magnesium, individually or in combination. Tums is an example of an antacid containing calcium carbonate. Aluminum and magnesium combinations include Maalox® and Mylanta®. Antacids are usually administered orally in liquid form or in tablet form. Side effects include acid rebound in products containing calcium carbonate, diarrhea in products containing magnesium, and constipation in products containing aluminum or calcium carbonate.

GI ulcers are open sores that occur within the stomach and duodenum where acid and pepsin are most active. Antiulcer drugs act as histamine receptor antagonists to reduce gastric secretion. Two common drugs, cimetidine (Tagamet®) and ranitidine (Zantac®), are used to treat duodenal ulcers and gastric ulcers. Famotidine (Pepcid®) has similar drug actions and is also used to treat these conditions.[9] Side effects are mild but may include diarrhea, dizziness, and headache.

Antidiarrheal agents include kaolin and pectin preparations (Kaopectate®), as well as diphenoxylate with atropine (Lomotil®) and loperamide (Imodium®). Kaopectate creates a drying effect by acting as an absorbant, whereas Lomotil and Imodium actually slow intestinal motility. Lomotil can produce anticholinergic side effects such as drying of secretions, blurred vision, urinary retention, and lethargy. Lomotil and Imodium both can cause abdominal distention, nausea, and vomiting. In direct contrast to the antidiarrheal drugs are the laxatives, which promote intestinal evacuation, and cathartics, which do the same, but also alter stool consistency. Drugs that fall into this category include bulk forming laxatives, stool softeners, and saline laxatives (Milk of Magnesia®). Saline laxatives should never be ingested on a regular basis, as prolonged use can cause electrolyte imbalance and CNS symptoms such as weakness, sedation, and confusion.

Antiemetics are drugs that decrease nausea and vomiting that occur postoperatively, with motion sickness, or as a result of other medical treatments, including cancer chemotherapy and radiation treatments. Phenothiazine (Phenergan®) can be prescribed for the treatment of nausea and vomiting after surgery. The antihistamine dimehydrinate (Dramamine®) is a popular choice for motion sickness. Side effects of antiemetics include sedation and drowsiness.

Drugs that affect the GI tract do not have a great impact on rehabilitation. Although many patients may have various GI disorders, pharmacological intervention works well to prevent any disruption in treatments. Antiemetic drugs can be useful to prevent the nausea and vomiting associated with chemotherapy in cancer patients, thus making their treatment experience more tolerable.

Pharmacology of the Endocrine System

The endocrine system is comprised of several glands situated throughout the body that release various hormones into the bloodstream. These hormones act to increase specific tissue activities in the body. Endocrine system drugs can be used as hormone replacement therapy and also to treat certain conditions such as chronic inflammation. These drugs can be naturally occurring hormones or they can be artificially produced synthetic hormones. Adrenal steroids, also known as corticosteroids, are used to relieve inflammation and reduce swelling. Corticosteroids can be administered orally, by injection, or topically. Steroid use can result in tissue breakdown, so caution must be used during rehabilitation when stressing muscles, bones, and joints so as to avoid further injury.

Pharmacological uses of female sex hormones include replacement therapy in cases of hormone deficiency, for oral contraception, to increase fertility, and therapy in certain types of cancer. Oral contraceptives are combinations of the hormones estrogen and progesterone that prevent pregnancy by inhibiting the release of follicle stimulating hormone (FSH) and luteinizing hormone (LH). Patients who are prescribed sex hormones should have their blood pressure monitored routinely because these drugs promote salt and water retention, which could lead to hypertension. Although androgens, or male sex hormones, can be used in cases of hormonal deficiencies, often these drugs are used illegally by athletes to increase muscle mass and improve athletic performance. Typically, men more often than women engage in anabolic steroid use. The athletic trainer should make the patient aware of the harmful effects of steroids, such as damage to the liver, cardiovascular system, and reproductive organs. Mood swings and aggressive behavior might be evident during rehabilitation. Being a source of accurate information about steroids may put the athletic trainer in a good position to discourage such use.

Diabetes mellitus is a condition characterized by abnormally high blood sugar levels due to a deficiency in the production and secretion of the hormone insulin. In juvenile diabetes, or type I diabetes, there is no insulin production by the body, necessitating the implementation of insulin therapy. Mature onset diabetes, or type II diabetes, is a result of a relative insulin deficiency, and usually occurs in older adults who are overweight. Oral hypoglycemic drugs (sulfonylurea drugs) are sometimes useful in the treatment of mature onset diabetes. These oral hypoglycemics actually enter the pancreas and promote the release of insulin. Type I diabetes requires the use of insulin, which must be administered by subcutaneous or IM injection. There are several conditions for which diabetics could seek clinical treatment, and most would be dealt with by a physical therapist. However, athletic trainers supervising exercise programs should be alert to the possibility of diabetic patients becoming hypoglycemic following physical exertion, especially if the patient skipped a meal prior to the rehabilitation session. It is suggested that a high-glucose snack be made available to alleviate the symptoms of hypoglycemia, which include confusion, fatigue, sweating, and nausea. IM injections can be absorbed rapidly, depending on the blood flow to the injection site. It is believed that joggers who inject insulin into their thigh could possibly experience a decrease in blood sugar, because running will increase blood flow to the leg.[18] This drop in blood sugar would not be expected if a different injection site, such as the arm or abdomen, had been selected prior to running.

Pharmacology of Infectious Diseases

Antibacterial drugs can be classified in two ways. Bacteriocidal drugs actually kill existing bacteria, while bacteriostatic drugs only inhibit the growth of new bacteria. There are several antibacterial drugs from which to choose, for it may be necessary to switch medications because some organisms can build up a resistance to certain drugs that have been used too long. Penicillins are common antibiotics used to treat many streptococcal and some staphylococcal infections. Penicillin has been used for the treatment of respiratory and intestinal infections, and also for the treatment of gonorrhea and syphilis. Erythromycin is one of the least toxic antibiotics and is used to treat respiratory tract infections and skin infections. Cephalosporins are broad spectrum antibiotics used to treat serious infections of the respiratory tract, skin, urinary tract, and bone and joints. Tetracyclines are another example of common antibiotics. There are several others.

Many of the bacterial drugs can cause hypersensitivity reactions. Skin rashes, itching, and respiratory difficulty are indications of these types of reactions and may be initially recognized by the athletic trainer. GI disturbances can also occur, but usually do not disrupt treatment sessions. Athletic trainers can help to decrease the spread of bacteria and other infections by washing their hands between patients, utilizing sterile techniques when caring for open wounds, and ensuring that whirlpools have been properly disinfected.

Antifungal drugs are usually administered topically or orally. These drugs are used to combat certain susceptible fungi. Fungal conditions such as tinea cruris (jock itch) and tinea pedis (athlete's foot) are typically treated with topical medications, but medications can be administered orally to treat tinea infections that do not respond to topical treatments. Athletic trainers may initially recognize fungal infections that had gone unnoticed by the patient. The athletic trainer should take the time to educate the patient in avoiding the spread of these infections. There are very few antiviral drugs. Acyclovir is a topical medication used to treat herpes simplex and herpes zoster. However, this drug does not kill the virus and only helps to relieve discomfort and shorten the healing time of existing lesions.

Chemotherapy of Cancer

Chemotherapy is defined as the use of drugs to kill cancer cells. Antineoplastic drugs inhibit tumor growth or cell reproduction. Antineoplastic drugs are extremely toxic, due to the fact that normal cells are destroyed along with cancer cells, because the drugs cannot differentiate between the two. Severe toxic and neurotoxic effects occur with the use of these cancer drugs. Cancer patients undergoing chemotherapy may not always be able to tolerate low intensity treatment sessions. Although athletic trainers may not typically deal with this population, they may have contact with these patients when asked to utilize modalities such as electrical stimulation to alleviate the patient's pain. It is important to be very understanding and psychologically supportive to these cancer patients.

SUMMARY

Athletic trainers in the clinical setting are likely to deal with patients who are taking pharmacological agents to treat the condition for which they are seeking treatment, or for another pre-existing condition. A basic knowledge of pharmacology allows the athletic trainer to understand how certain medications may affect rehabilitation, and to also recognize that rehabilitation may alter the pharmaceutical effects of certain drugs. By understanding the interaction between pharmacology and rehabilitation, the athletic trainer can appropriately schedule patients and effectively prescribe rehabilitation programs based on the patient's response to their medication.

Study Questions

1. Define pharmacology and discuss its relationship to clinical athletic training.
2. Explain how drug nomenclature is used to identify the different names of individual medications.
3. Differentiate between pharmacodynamics and pharmacokinetics as they relate to the principles of pharmacology.
4. What are the major routes of drug administration? What are the advantages and disadvantages of each mechanism of delivery?
5. Consider a patient who is taking medication for hypertension, what concerns would you have prior to the development of an exercise program for this individual? What concerns would you have for someone taking medications for each of the following conditions?
   - Epilepsy
   - Acute low back pain
   - Depression
   - Muscle spasm
   - Pulmonary edema
   - Asthma
   - GI ulcer
   - Diabetes mellitus
6. What are common methods by which a clinical athletic trainer can obtain information regarding certain medications?

References

1. Asperheim MK. *Pharmacologic Basis of Patient Care*. 5th ed. Philadelphia, Pa: W.B. Saunders Company; 1985.
2. Parish P. *The Doctors and Patients Handbook of Medicines and Drugs*. New York, NY: Alfred A. Knopf, Inc.; 1977.
3. Ciccone CD. Introduction: Pharmacology. *Phys Ther*. 1995;75:342.
4. Ciccone CD. Basic pharmacokinetics and the potential effects of physical therapy interventions on pharmacokinetic variables. *Phys Ther*. 1995;75:343-351.
5. Ciccone CD. *Pharmacology in Rehabilitation*. 2nd ed. Philadelphia, Pa: F.A. Davis Company; 1996.
6. Witlers W, Venturelli, Hanson G. *Drugs and Society*. 3rd ed. Boston, Mass: Jones and Bartlett Publishers, Inc.; 1992.

7. Swonger AK, Matejski MP. *Nursing Pharmacology*. Boston, Mass: Scott, Foresman, and Co.; 1988.

8. Clayton BD, Stock YN, Squire JE. *Squire's Basic Pharmacology for Nurses*. 8th ed. St. Louis, Mo: The C. V. Mosby Co.; 1985.

9. Woodrow R. *Essentials of Pharmacology for Health Occupations*. 2nd ed. Albany, NY: Delmar Publishers, Inc.; 1992.

10. Whitehill WR, Wright KE, Robinson JB. Guidelines for dispensing medications. *J Athl Train*. 1992;27:20-22.

11. Skidmore-Roth L. *Mosby's Nursing Drug Reference*. St. Louis, Mo: Mosby-Year Book, Inc.; 1996.

12. Hitner H, Nagle BT. *Basic Pharmacology for Health Occupations*. Indianapolis, Ind: The Bobbs-Merrill Company, Inc.; 1980.

13. *Physicians' Desk Reference*. 49th ed. Montvale, NJ: Medical Economics Data Production Company; 1995.

14. *Physicians' Desk Reference for Nonprescription Drugs*. 15th ed. Montvale, NJ: Medical Economics Data Production Company; 1994.

15. Benet LZ, Mitchell JR, Sheiner LB. Introduction. In: Gilman AG, Rall TW, Nies AS, Taylor P, eds. *The Pharmacological Basis of Therapeutics*. 8th ed. New York, NY: Pergamon Press, Inc.; 1990.

16. Baer CL. General Pharmacology: Introduction. In: Baer CL, Williams BR, eds. *Clinical Pharmacology and Nursing*. Springhouse, Pa: Springhouse Publishing Co.; 1988.

17. Jacob LS. *Pharmacology*. 2nd ed. New York, NY: John Wiley & Sons, Inc.; 1987.

18. Benet LZ, Mitchell JR, Sheiner LB. Pharmacokinetics: The Dynamics of Drug Absorption, Distribution and Elimination. In: Gilman AG, Rall TW, Nies AS, Taylor P, eds. *The Pharmacological Basis of Therapeutics*. 8th ed. New York, NY: Pergamon Press, Inc.; 1990.

19. Arnheim DD, Prentice WE. *Principles of Athletic Training*. 8th ed. St. Louis, Mo: MosbyYear Book, Inc.; 1993.

CHAPTER
20

Outcomes Assessment in Athletic Training

Michael A. Keirns, PhD, ATC, PT, CSCS
Lyle Knudson, EdD
Keith J. Webster, MA, ATC

OBJECTIVES

Upon completion of this chapter, the student will be able to accomplish the following:

1. Discuss how outcomes can be used by patients, athletic trainers, and payers to measure the effects of an intervention

2. Be familiar with the major categories of outcomes studies and the functions of each

3. Define efficacy, effectiveness, quality of care, and quality assessment, and recognize the relationships among them

4. Describe the goals of the Athletic Training Outcomes Assessment study and explain how the data obtained can be utilized

5. Recognize the important role that the athletic trainer plays in outcomes assessment studies

O utcomes assessment is a systematic method used for measuring the effects of an intervention. In the field of athletic training, changes in the health status of people with activity-related injuries as a result of the care provided by athletic trainers are being measured. These data will provide patients with valuable information as they make decisions regarding appropriate providers for their health care needs. Athletic trainers will be better able to define their effectiveness, scope of practice, and educational objectives. These data will support treatment and rehabilitation protocols and allow athletic trainers to develop expected outcomes. The most cost-effective strategy can also be determined from data analysis and outcomes management, which is important to those who pay for health care.

TYPES OF OUTCOMES STUDIES

Three major categories of outcomes studies are: 1) clinical outcomes, 2) functional outcomes, and 3) patient satisfaction. *Clinical outcome studies* typically measure the results of physician intervention in terms of mortality and morbidity under carefully controlled and specifically defined circumstances, providing clinicians with new ways of managing disease processes and prolonging meaningful life. *Functional outcomes studies* measure the patient's physical, mental, and social function as well as the patient's perception of pain and other quality of life factors. *Patient satisfaction* is measured in terms of the patient's assessment of the care provided and its effect on his or her overall well-being.

Outcomes studies address the change in status of the patient's health over time and the related cost of the resources utilized to care for that patient. Cost may not in itself be considered a patient outcome; however, consumers (patients) and payers of health care are demanding to know the value of the care. Determining that value requires knowledge of all the processes or steps involved in providing health care services.

Health care research addresses the efficacy, the effectiveness, variations in the delivery process, and the quality of care. *Efficacy* refers to "the probability of benefit to individuals in a defined population from a medical technology applied for a given medical problem under ideal conditions of use."[1] Randomized clinical trials provide the best method for establishing efficacy. One example is to study new drugs or drug treatment protocols. However, efficacious techniques in athletic training are not easily established because of a general lack of randomized clinical trials. Thus, athletic trainers usually rely on expert judgment. *Effectiveness* is the "extent to which benefits achievable under optimal conditions of care are actually achieved in clinical practice."[2] Studying or measuring the efficacy of a technique and its appropriate use is most difficult in an allied health setting. Allied health services address the alleviation or amelioration of symptoms rather than the corrective or curative measures provided by medical practitioners; thus, attention is given to functional and quality of life issues.

USES OF OUTCOMES STUDIES

Outcomes management lacks the purposeful randomization of a clinical trial, but it would generate information about the results of the natural, seemingly random variations in practice style. It differs from a clinical trial in another important way: With outcomes management, standards and outcome measures would be constantly subject to modification based on the results of analysis and feedback.[3]

Therefore, any resultant standards or benchmarks realized from a broad national study are not concrete and unchanging. Rather, standards become part of a continuum that is measured and improved over time. By studying the specific nature of athletic training outcomes, athletic trainers address the variations in the overall health care delivery process. The question to be answered by all health care providers is "do we provide appropriate and effective care to our patients?" Athletic trainers find themselves in a unique situation when trying to address this issue accurately. By nature, athletic trainers treat and manage injuries that are caused by a specific activity, usually with few or no other co-morbid factors or underlying pathology and without other health care providers giving care aside from the supervising physician who gives input and direction. Thus, athletic trainers can isolate the specific role they play as a health care provider to the patient population by studying and measuring the outcome of the care they provide.

Quality of Care

Quality of care can best be described as "that component of the difference between efficacy and effectiveness that can be attributed to care providers, taking account of the environment in which they work. 'Quality assessment' . . . is the measurement of the technical and interpersonal aspects of medical care."[4] Quality of care affects clinical outcomes, functional outcomes, and patient satisfaction.

Quality of care can now be addressed more objectively by outcomes studies than by other less precise techniques, such as reviews of medical records. A complete and accurate description of quality assessment must include information beyond that contained in the patients' charts. For example, the provider's treatment recommendations for a particular condition may be influenced by his or her experience, as well as the ability to work within a health care framework defined by a third party. The patient's motivation to recover may be affected by personality and coping skills.

When addressing quality issues, one very important aspect is the patient's perception of quality. Therefore, the provider may report a poor clinical outcome because a particular patient cannot run a marathon, when in fact the patient is satisfied that the personal goal of functioning in his or her physical environment (i.e., activities of daily living) was achieved. A clinician must always consider the patient's own value system. Using outcomes analysis, the practicality of patients' goals and expectations can be addressed more clearly. Benchmarks derived from outcomes analysis can be useful in defining quality standards. Applying the results of outcomes-generated benchmarks to cost models can also help define economic quality of care.

If conducted efficiently by a valid instrument, outcomes assessment can identify the relationships among quality of care, benchmarks, and the patient's own value system, and can determine if these factors are being addressed correctly. The economics of health care is a driving force behind outcomes studies. Government officials and third-party payers are looking at outcomes as one way to monitor and control medical expenses. The federal government's creation of the Agency for Health Care, Policy, and Research in 1989 reflected the government's interest in reviewing and determining which medical treatments produce the best and most cost-effective patient outcomes. The Agency's medical treatment effectiveness program funds research to determine which clinical strategies contribute the most to maintaining health, functional independence, and patient satisfaction.

Other research projects include patient outcomes research teams, or PORTs. For these interdisciplinary studies, meta-analysis of existing data and of new interventions are included in the evaluation of the effects of interventions on patient outcomes. The second generation PORT II projects have continued to put the patient first while establishing direct links between practice and outcomes. Attempts are also being made to study direct comparisons of alternative clinical strategies.

MEASURING OUTCOMES

Choosing the instrument that would most accurately measure athletic training outcomes was a formidable challenge. Early versions of "general health status" and "quality of life" instruments (e.g., Medical Outcome Study [MOS], Health Status Questionnaire [HSQ]) were very time-consuming and applicable to clinical trials but were not practical in the athletic training setting. Abbreviated versions (e.g., Short Form 36 [SF-36]) were developed and provided good measures of general health outcomes suitable for evaluating chronic illness and injuries, but they were essentially irrelevant for evaluating the treatment and rehabilitation for acute activity-related injuries most often treated by athletic trainers.

Orthopedists developed instruments (e.g., Lysholm Knee Rating System) that focused mainly on activities of daily living and less on sports and recreation functions of the active population that are treated by athletic trainers.

The Athletic Training Outcomes Assessment

In 1995, through the efforts of its governmental affairs committee, the National Athletic Trainers' Association (NATA) formed a task force to address the issues that involved reimbursement of athletic training services, which became known as the NATA Reimbursement Advisory Group. The task force, chaired by Marjorie Albohm, recognized the need to develop an outcomes instrument for athletic trainers. NATA commissioned BIO*Analysis Systems to develop such an instrument. Following formal research and the development of procedures, the Athletic Training Outcomes Assessment (ATOA) was produced. This instrument integrates the individual strengths of the previously developed general medical outcomes assessment instruments with new and innovative approaches. The ATOA is applicable to a broad range of injury locations and diagnoses. It offers multidimensional definitions of outcomes, links specific treatments with outcomes, and provides direct assessment of the procedures in an effort to reduce the time and cost of the treatment. The ATOA data are specific to injuries, treatments, effective variables, risk factors, and outcomes expectations (Figure 20-1 represents an excerpt of ATOA).

The ATOA study should help athletic trainers to improve reimbursement, provide professional self-assessment, create benchmarks, and apply costing models to their services. Initially, reimbursement was the driving force behind conducting the national outcomes study. Payment sources, such as third-party payers, insurance companies, and managed care administrators, wanted to know the results of the care provided by athletic trainers,

ATHLETIC TRAINING OUTCOMES ASSESSMENT©
TO BE COMPLETED AT INITIAL ENCOUNTER

Site–Athletic Trainer Code _____   Patient Name_____ Age ____ Sex ____
(for site use only)

Site Type _____
1. Sports Medicine Clinic
2. Clinic–High School/College
3. High School Training Room
4. College/University Training Room
5. Professional Training Room
6. Industrial Setting

Referring Source _____
1. Self
2. Coach/Supervisor
3. Insurer
4. Primary Care Physician/Generalist
5. Orthopedic Physician/Specialist

Payer _____
1. Medicaid
2. Medicare
3. Managed Care
4. Workers' Compensation
5. Champus (government/military)
6. Private Insurance
7. Institution
8. Patient

TO BE COMPLETED BY ATHLETIC TRAINER AT INITIAL EVALUATION

Duration Between Injury/Surgery and Beginning of Athletic Training Treatments _____ days
(Put 0 if treatments begin on the same day as the injury/surgery.)

Location of Injury/Surgery _____
(Give only the one most primary location. If another injury, identify as a Comorbid Factor.)

1. toe(s)	4. lower leg	7. hip	10. abdomen	13. cervical	16. arm	19. wrist
2. foot	5. knee	8. pelvis	11. lumbar	14. head	17. elbow	20. hand
3. ankle	6. thigh	9. groin	12. thorax	15. shoulder	18. forearm	21. finger(s)

Type of Injury _____
(Give only the one most primary injury. If another injury at another location, identify as a Comorbid Factor.)

1. joint dysfunction	9. strain; grade III	17. skin/wound infection	25. fracture
2. joint degeneration	10. sprain; grade I	18. bursitis	26. avulsion
3. joint hypomobility	11. sprain; grade II	19. musculo-tendonous injury	27. neurologic disease

TO BE COMPLETED BY PATIENT AT INTAKE AND DISCHARGE

Patient–Your responses to this questionnaire will help your athletic trainer and this clinic determine rehabilitation outcomes for specific medical conditions in response to specific treatments. This will help us optimize our treatment services to you and other patients. Your responses will be kept confidential and will not affect your care in any way. Thanks for your assistance.

AT INTAKE   **AT DISCHARGE**

Instructions–Please rate your current capacities specific to the injury for which you will receive, or have received, treatments. Please answer all questions as best you can, even if some of the questions seem somewhat irrelevant to you. Circle the appropriate response according to the (0 1 2 3 4) scale; 0 - critical problem, 1 - severe problem, 2 - moderate problem, 3 - minor problem, 4 - no problem.

INTAKE CRITICAL / SEVERE / MODERATE / MINOR / NO PROBLEM	Item	DISCHARGE CRITICAL / SEVERE / MODERATE / MINOR / NO PROBLEM
0 1 2 3 4	**Work Activities**–lifting/lowering, holding/handling, carrying, pushing/pulling, bending over, squatting/stooping, kneeling, crawling, reaching, turning/pivoting, gripping/pinching, fingering	0 1 2 3 4
0 1 2 3 4	**Sports/Recreation/Wellness Activities**–running, jumping, throwing, catching, kicking, swinging, withstanding impacts, weightlifting, specific sport/recreation/wellness activity	0 1 2 3 4
0 1 2 3 4	**Movement**–getting into desired positions, range of motion, speed of motion, bilateral differences (e.g., limping), need for support device	0 1 2 3 4

Figure 20-1. Excerpt from the Athletic Training Outcomes Assessment forms. Reprinted with permission from BIO*Analysis Systems.

a question being asked of virtually all allied health care providers who are currently receiving reimbursement for their services. When determining reimbursement, payers look at outcomes data, scope of practice, and education and credentialing requirements. In those states with no legislation regarding athletic training or with laws that restrict an athletic trainer's ability to receive reimbursement, outcomes could become vitally important in providing further proof of the quality of the national credentialing process in terms that payers will understand. Outcomes can also be used to support new legislation or revise existing laws.

Outcomes data also allow athletic trainers to examine what they do more objectively than ever before. Athletic trainers take pride in working long, hard hours; however, this admirable work ethic does not automatically ensure the best outcomes. Typically, athletic trainers use all appropriate modalities available during several daily treatment periods for an injured athlete. Outcome then is measured by the athlete's ability to return to the next contest, a bottom line standard that will always be important. However, outcomes analysis provides information regarding the best utilization of treatment and rehabilitation resources, which allows athletic trainers to become more efficient and productive during the process used to reach the bottom line standard.

The use of outcomes data can also help validate the credentialing process, giving curriculum directors another tool to evaluate their education programs. Additional uses of outcomes data will become apparent as more data are collected over time.

The creation and modification of benchmarks are by-products of outcomes data analysis as discussed earlier. The benchmarks suggested by analysis of data and outcomes assessment are not rigid laws to be followed blindly but are to be modified as athletic trainers show proof that what they do is truly effective and efficient. In addition, every health care profession today is charged with demonstrating or establishing expected outcomes from the care they provide.

Some athletic trainers say that if economic factors are not integrated with outcomes data, then the results will not fully and effectively convey cost-effectiveness. The Reimbursement Advisory Group is investigating various costing models that best reflect the services provided by athletic trainers. Eventually, outcomes data will be applied to a model that will accurately measure the costs associated with the delivery of athletic training services.

The ATOA evaluates the outcomes from the use of athletic training treatment modalities to numerous injury categories at all body locations. The athletic trainer records the site type, referring source, and payer. The ATOA takes into account various affective variables that can influence patient responses (e.g., patient's age and sex; location, type, and severity of injury; number, duration, and frequency of treatments; risk factors [duration between injury and beginning of treatments, previous episode, co-morbid factors]). The ATOA is targeted at sport-, recreation-, and work-related injuries and measures general health status; specific medical conditions; activities of daily living function; work activities function; and sports, recreation, and wellness function improvements; and various physical (i.e., movement, strength and power, endurance, motor abilities, body structure, sensation) and psychosocial outcomes. At discharge, the patient completes a self-assessment of the treatment and the athletic trainer rates the athlete's and the coach's or supervisor's compliance. The Assessment uses the patient's and athletic trainer's pre- and posttreatment ratings of each functional, physical, and satisfaction and compliance variable in 13 queries to define the patient's outcomes.

The ATOA involves simple central tendency (means and standard deviations) and relational (multivariate correlations) statistics expressed in numerical and bar graph form in quarterly reports. The analyses and reports for all injury locations, injury categories, and treatments are in three parts: 1) absolute outcomes that describe an athletic trainer's or site's outcomes independent of other athletic trainers or sites in the ATOA national database; 2) relative outcomes that compare the outcomes of the athletic trainer or site with the ATOA results of all the athletic trainers and sites; and 3) special outcomes that relate each affective variable and risk factor to the outcomes. The ATOA was used for a National Athletic Trainers Association-funded study to record outcomes from 100 sites over a 3-year period. BIO*Analysis provided the analysis and produced quarterly reports.

SUMMARY

For outcomes assessment studies to be most effective, they must be incorporated into the athletic trainer's everyday documentation process. Students need to understand and continue the process of evaluating outcomes to allow the profession to evolve. Working harder does not always produce better outcomes. Athletic trainers need to expand their knowledge and test new approaches in their practice to achieve better outcomes and to become more efficient. Such advances will help to further establish the value of an athletic trainer's processes and outcomes.

Study Questions

1. List and describe the three major categories of outcomes studies. What do each of the three types of outcomes studies measure?
2. List three uses of outcomes assessment data in athletic training.
3. Identify three goals of the Athletic Training Outcomes Assessment study.
4. What are the differences between outcomes management and clinical trials?
5. Differentiate between quality care and quality assessment.
6. How would you define the athletic trainer's role in establishing effective outcomes studies?

References

1. U.S. Congress Office of Technology Assessment. The concepts of efficacy and safety. In: *Assessing the Efficacy and Safety of Medical Technologies*. Washington, DC: U.S. Government Printing Office; 1978:16.

2. Williamson JW. Basing quality assurance on the outcomes of care. In: *Assessing and Improving Health Care Outcomes: The Health Accounting Approach to Quality Assurance*. Cambridge, Mass: Ballinger Publishing Company; 1978:10.

3. Ellwood PM. Shattuck Lecture—Outcomes management. A technology of patient experience. *New Engl J Med.* 1988;318:1549-1556.

4. Brook RH, Lohr KN. Efficacy, effectiveness, variations, and quality: Boundary-crossing research. *Medical Care.* 1985;23:710-711.

Suggested Readings

Abanobi OC. Content validity in the assessment of health status. *Health Values*. 1986;10:37-43.

American Medical Association. *Guides to the Evaluation of Permanent Impairment*. 4th ed. Chicago, Ill: American Medical Association; 1993.

Bartko JJ, Carpenter WT Jr. On the methods and theory of reliability. *J Nerv Ment Dis*. 1976;163:307-317.

Berwick DM, Murphy JM, Goldman PA, Ware JE Jr, Barsky AJ, Weinstein MC. Performance of a five-item mental health screening test. *Med Care*. 1991;29:169-176.

Bloom BS. Does it work? The outcomes of medical interventions. *Int J Technol Assess Health Care*. 1990;6:326-332.

Dodds TA, Martin DP, Stolov WC, Deyo RA. A validation of the functional independence measurement and its performance among rehabilitation inpatients. *Arch Phy Med Rehab*. 1993;74:531-536.

Eazell DE. Demonstrating cost savings through functional gains. *Rehab Mngmt*. 1992; Aug-Sept:137-139.

Ellingham CT, Abeln SH. Quality assurance and total quality management. In: Stewart DL, Abeln SH, eds. *Documenting Functional Outcomes in Physical Therapy*. St. Louis, Mo: C.V. Mosby; 1993.

Esposto L. Applying functional outcome assessment to Medicare documentation. In: Stewart DL, Abeln SH, eds. *Documenting Functional Outcomes in Physical Therapy*. St. Louis, Mo: C.V. Mosby; 1993.

Evans RL, Haselkorn JK, Bishop DS, Hendricks RD. Characteristics of hospital patients receiving medical rehabilitation: an exploratory outcome comparison. *Arch Phys Med Rehab*. 1991;72:685-689.

Fuhrer MJ. *Rehabilitation Outcomes: Analysis and Measurement*. Baltimore, Md: Paul H. Brookes Publishing Co.; 1987.

Golden WE. Health status measurement. Implementation strategies. *Med Care*. 1992;30(5;suppl):MS187-MS195.

Heinemann AW, Linacre JM, Wright BD, Hamilton BB, Granger C. Prediction of rehabilitation outcomes with disability measures. *Arch Phys Med Rehab*. 1994;75:133-143.

Jette AM. Using health-related quality of life measures in physical therapy outcomes research. *Phys Ther*. 1993;73:528-537.

Jette AM, Davies AR, Cleary PD, et al. The Functional Status Questionnaire: reliability and validity when used in primary care. *J Gen Int Med*. 1986;1:143-149.

Laughlin JA, Granger CV, Hamilton BB. Outcomes measurement in medical rehabilitation. *Rehab Mngmt*. 1992;Dec-Jan:57-58.

Law M. Evaluating activities of daily living: directions for the future. *Am J Occup Ther*. 1993;47:233-237.

Roland M, Morris R. A study of the natural history of back pain; Part 1:development of a reliable and sensitive measure of disability in low-back pain. *Spine*. 1983;8:141-144.

Saliva ME, Mayfield MD, Weissman NW. Patient outcomes research teams and the Agency for Health Care Policy and research. *Health Serv Res*. 1990;25:697-708.

Schwartz JS, Lurie N. Assessment of medical outcomes:new opportunities for achieving a long sought-after objective. *Int J Technol Assess Health Care*. 1990;6:333-339.

Simborg DW, Whiting-O'Keefe QE. Evaluation methodology for ambulatory care information systems. *Med Care*. 1982;20:255-265.

Sisk JE. Introduction to measuring health care effectiveness. *Int J Technol Assess Health Care*. 1990;6:181-182.

Steinwachs DM. Application of health status assessment measures in policy research. *Med Care*. 1989;27(3; suppl):S12-S26.

Stewart AL, Hays RD, Ware JE Jr. The MOS Short form general health survey. Reliability and validity in a patient population. *Med Care*. 1988;26:724-735.

Taulbee P. Outcomes management: buying value and cutting costs. *Bus Health*. 1991;9(3):28-39.

Tegner Y, Lysholm J. Rating systems in the evaluation of knee ligament injuries. *Clin Orthop*. 1985;198:43-49.

Tugwell P, Bombardier C, Buchanan WW, Goldsmith CH, Grace E, Hanna B. The MACTAR Patient Preference Disability Questionnaire—an individualized functional priority approach for assessing improvement in physical disability in clinical trials in rheumatoid arthritis. *J Rheum*. 1987;14:446-451.

Verbrugge LM, Lepkowski JM, Imanaka V. Comorbidity and its impact on disability. *Milbank Q*. 1989;67:450-485.

Ware JE Jr, Hays RD. Methods for measuring patient satisfaction with specific medical encounters. *Med Care*. 1988;26:393-402.

Ware JE Jr, Shelbourne CD. The MOS 36-item Short form health survey questionnaire (SF-36);I. Conceptual framework and item selection. *Med Care*. 1992;30:473-481.

Wasson J, Keller A, Rubenstein L, Hays R, Nelson E, Johnson D, The Dartmouth Primary Care COOP Project. Benefits and obstacles of health status assessment in ambulatory settings. *Med Care*. 1992;30(5;supp):MS42-MS49.

Wennberg JE. Improving the medical decision-making process. *Health Aff-Millwood*. 1988;7:99-106.

Wyszewianski L. Quality of care:past achievements and future challenges. *Inquiry*. 1988;25:13-22.

National Athletic Trainers' Association Mission Statement

The mission of the National Athletic Trainers' Association is to enhance the quality of health care for the physically active and advance the profession of athletic training through education and research in the prevention, evaluation, management, and rehabilitation of injuries.

Reprinted with permission from the NATA.

APPENDIX

B

National Athletic Trainers' Association Code of Ethics

PREAMBLE

The Code of Ethics of the National Athletic Trainers' Association has been written to make the membership aware of the principles of ethical behavior that should be followed in the practice of athletic training. The primary goal of the Code is the assurance of high quality health care. The Code presents aspirational standards of behavior that all members should strive to achieve.

The principles cannot be expected to cover all specific situations that may be encountered by the practicing athletic trainer, but should be considered representative of the spirit with which athletic trainers should make decisions. The principles are written generally and the circumstances of a situation will determine the interpretation and application of a given principle and of the Code as a whole. Whenever there is a conflict between the Code and legality, the laws prevail. The guidelines set forth in this Code are subject to continued review and revision as the athletic training profession develops and changes.

PRINCIPLE 1: MEMBERS SHALL RESPECT THE RIGHTS, WELFARE, AND DIGNITY OF ALL INDIVIDUALS.

1.1. Members shall neither practice nor condone discrimination on the basis of race, creed, national origin, sex, age, handicap, disease entity, social status, financial status, or religious affiliation.

1.2. Members shall be committed to providing competent care consistent with both the requirements and the limitations of their profession.

1.3. Members shall preserve the confidentiality of privileged information and shall not release such information to a third party not involved in the patient's care unless the person consents to such release or release is permitted or required by law.

PRINCIPLE 2: MEMBERS SHALL COMPLY WITH THE LAWS AND REGULATIONS GOVERNING THE PRACTICE OF ATHLETIC TRAINING.

2.1. Members shall comply with applicable local, state, and federal laws and institutional guidelines.

2.2. Members shall be familiar with and adhere to all National Athletic Trainers' Association guidelines and ethical standards.

2.3. Members are encouraged to report illegal or unethical practice pertaining to athletic training to the appropriate person or authority.

2.4. Members shall avoid substance abuse and, when necessary, seek rehabilitation for chemical dependency.

PRINCIPLE 3: MEMBERS SHALL ACCEPT RESPONSIBILITY FOR THE EXERCISE OF SOUND JUDGMENT.

3.1. Members shall not misrepresent in any manner, either directly or indirectly, their skills, training, professional credentials, identity, or services.

3.2. Members shall provide only those services for which they are qualified via education and/or experience and by pertinent legal regulatory process.

3.3. Members shall provide services, make referrals, and seek compensation only for those services that are necessary.

PRINCIPLE 4: MEMBERS SHALL MAINTAIN AND PROMOTE HIGH STANDARDS IN THE PROVISION OF SERVICES.

4.1. Members shall recognize the need for continuing education and participate in various types of educational activities that enhance their skills and knowledge.

4.2. Members who have the responsibility for employing and evaluating the performance of other staff members shall fulfill such responsibility in a fair, considerate, and equitable manner, on the basis of clearly enunciated criteria.

4.3. Members who have the responsibility for evaluating the performance of employees, supervisors, or students are encouraged to share evaluations with them and allow them the opportunity to respond to those evaluations.

4.4. Members shall educate those whom they supervise in the practice of athletic training with regard to the Code of Ethics and encourage their adherence to it.

4.5. Whenever possible, members are encouraged to participate and support others in the conduct and communication of research and educational activities that may contribute knowledge for improved patient care, patient or student education, and the growth of athletic training as a profession.

4.6. When members are researchers or educators, they are responsible for maintaining and promoting ethical conduct in research and educational activities.

PRINCIPLE 5: MEMBERS SHALL NOT ENGAGE IN ANY FORM OF CONDUCT THAT CONSTITUTES A CONFLICT OF INTEREST OR THAT ADVERSELY REFLECTS ON THE PROFESSION.

5.1. The private conduct of the member is a personal matter to the same degree as is any other person's except when such conduct promises the fulfillment of professional responsibilities.

5.2. Members of the National Athletic Trainers' Association and others serving on the Association's committees or acting as consultants shall not use, directly or by implication, the Association's name or logo or their affiliation with the Association in the endorsement of products or services.

5.3. Members shall not place financial gain above the welfare of the patient being treated and shall not participate in any arrangement that exploits the patient.

5.4. Members may seek remuneration for their services that is commensurate with their services and in compliance with applicable law.

Reprinted with permission from National Athletic Trainers' Assocation Code of Ethics. *NATA News.* November 1993:10-11.

Clinical/ Industrial/ Corporate Athletic Trainers' Committee Position Statement

An increasing number of individuals participate in organized and recreational sports, leading to an increase in sports-related injuries. This increase, in turn, has led to significant growth in the number of sports-injury treatment settings. The services provided to individuals in these settings are rendered by practitioners from a variety of disciplines. Among these practitioners are Certified Athletic Trainers.

The Clinical/Industrial/Corporate Athletic Trainers' Committee of the National Athletic Trainers' Association adopts the following position:

1. The services provided to physically active people should always be in keeping with their needs and best interests.
2. Certified Athletic Trainers should not misrepresent themselves to the public.
3. Certified Athletic Trainers provide athletic training services in accordance with the Domains of Athletic Training and the laws of the jurisdiction in which they practice. The

domains of Athletic Training are the following:
- Prevention of injuries to the physically active
- Recognition, evaluation, and immediate care of injuries to the physically active
- Rehabilitation and reconditioning of injuries to the physically active
- Health care administration
- Professional development and responsibility

4. The Certified Athletic Trainer shall provide services under the direction of the physician of record.

Reprinted with permission from the NATA.

Blood Borne Pathogens Guidelines for Athletic Trainers

The NATA recognizes that blood borne pathogens such as HIV, HBV, and HCV present many complex issues for athletic trainers, athletic administrators, and others involved with the care and training of athletes. As the primary health care profession involved with the physically active, it is important for athletic trainers to be aware of these issues. The NATA therefore offers the following guidelines and information concerning the management of blood borne pathogen-related issues in the context of athletics and settings in which the physically active are involved.

It is essential to remember, however, that the medical, legal, and professional knowledge, standards, and requirements concerning blood borne pathogens are changing and evolving constantly and vary, in addition, from place to place and from setting to setting. The guidance provided in these guidelines must not, therefore, be taken to represent national standards applicable to members of the NATA. Rather, the guidance here is intended to highlight issues, problems, and potential approaches to (or management of) those problems that NATA members can consider when developing their own policies with respect to management of these issues.

ATHLETIC PARTICIPATION

Decisions regarding the participation of athletes infected with blood borne pathogens in athletic competitions should be made on an individual basis, following the standard or appropriate procedures generally followed with respect to health-related participation questions, and taking into account only those factors that are directly relevant to the health and rights of the athlete, the other participants in the competition, and the other constituencies with interests in the competition, the athletic program, the athletes, and the sponsoring schools or organizations.

The following are examples of factors that are appropriate in many settings to the decision-making process:

1. The current health of the athlete
2. The nature and intensity of the athlete's training
3. The physiological effects of the athletic competition
4. The potential risks of the infection being transmitted
5. The desires of the athlete
6. The administrative and legal needs of the competitive program

EDUCATION OF THE PHYSICALLY ACTIVE

In a rapidly changing medical, social, and legal environment, educational information concerning blood borne pathogens is of particular importance. The athletic trainer should play a role with respect to the creation and dissemination of educational information that is appropriate to and particularized with respect to that athletic trainer's position and responsibilities.

Athletic trainers who are responsible for developing educational programs with respect to blood borne pathogens should provide appropriate information concerning the following:

1. The risk of transmission of infection during competition
2. The risk of transmission or infection generally
3. The availability of HIV testing
4. The availability of HBV testing and vaccinations

Athletic trainers who have educational program responsibility should extend education efforts to include those, such as athletes' families and communities, who are directly or indirectly affected by the presence of blood borne pathogens in athletic competitions.

All education activities should, of course, be limited to those within athletic trainers' scope of practice and competence, be within their job descriptions or other relevant roles, and be undertaken with the cooperation and/or consent of appropriate personnel, such as team physicians, coaches, athletic directors, school or institutional counsel, and school and community leaders.

THE ATHLETIC TRAINER AND BLOOD BORNE PATHOGENS AT ATHLETIC EVENTS

The risk of blood borne pathogen transmission at athletic events is directly associated with contact with blood or other body fluids. Athletic trainers who have responsibility for overseeing events at which such contact is possible should use appropriate preventative measures and be prepared to administer appropriate treatment, consistent with the requirements and restrictions of their jobs and local, state, and federal law.

In most cases, these measures will include the following:

1. Pre-event care and covering of existing wounds, cuts, and abrasions
2. Provision of the necessary or usual equipment and supplies for compliance with universal precautions, including, for example, latex gloves, biohazard containers, disinfectants, bleach solutions, antiseptics, and sharps containers
3. Early recognition and control of a bleeding athlete, including measures such as appropriate cleaning and covering procedures, or changing of blood-saturated clothes
4. Requiring all athletes to report all wounds immediately
5. Insistence that universal precaution guidelines be followed at all times in the management of acute blood exposure
6. Appropriate cleaning and disposal policies and procedures for contaminated areas or equipment
7. Appropriate policies with respect to the delivery of life-saving techniques in the absence of protective equipment
8. Post-event management including, as appropriate, reevaluation, coverage of wounds, cuts, and abrasions
9. Appropriate policy development, including incorporation, with necessary legal and administrative assistance, of existing Occupational Safety and Health Administration (OSHA) and other legal guidelines and conference or school rules and regulations

STUDENT ATHLETIC TRAINER EDUCATION

NATA encourages appropriate education by and involvement of the student athletic trainer in educational efforts involving blood borne pathogens. These efforts and programs will vary significantly based on local needs, requirements, resources, and policies.

At the secondary school level, education efforts should include items such as the following:

1. Education and training in the use of universal precautions and first aid for wounds
2. Education regarding the risks of transmission/infection from the participants for whom they care
3. Education on the availability of HIV testing
4. Education on the availability of HBV vaccinations and testing
5. Education of parents or guardians regarding the students' risk of infection

At the college or university level, education efforts should include items such as those listed above and, as appropriate, the following:

1. Education in basic and clinical science of blood borne pathogens
2. Discussions regarding the ethical and social issues related to blood borne pathogens
3. The importance of prevention programs
4. Education concerning the signs and symptoms of HBV and HIV, as consistent with the scope of practice of the athletic profession and state and local law

UNIVERSAL PRECAUTIONS AND OSHA REGULATIONS

Athletic trainers should, consistent with their job descriptions and the time and legal requirements and limitations of their jobs and professions, inform themselves and other affected and interested parties of the relevant legal guidance and requirements affecting the handling and treatment of blood borne pathogens.

Athletic trainers cannot be expected to practice law or medicine, and efforts with respect to compliance with these guidelines and requirements must be commensurate with the athletic trainer's profession and professional requirements. It may be appropriate for athletic trainers to keep copies of the Center for Disease Control (CDC) and OSHA regulations and guidelines available for their own and others' use.

MEDICAL RECORDS AND CONFIDENTIALITY

The security, record-keeping, and confidentiality requirements and concerns that relate to athletes' medical records generally apply equally to those portions of athletes' medical records that concern blood borne pathogens.

Because social stigma is sometimes attached to individuals infected with blood borne pathogens, athletic trainers should pay particular care to the security, record-keeping, and confidentiality requirements that govern the medical records for which they have a professional obligation to see, use, keep, interpret, record, update, or otherwise handle.

Security, record-keeping, and confidentiality procedures should be maintained with respect to the records of other athletic trainers, employees, student athletic trainers, and athletes to the extent that the athletic trainer has responsibility for these records.

THE INFECTED ATHLETIC TRAINER

An athletic trainer infected with a blood borne pathogen should practice the profession of athletic training taking into account all professionally, medically, and legally relevant issues raised by the infection. Depending on individual circumstances, the infected athletic trainer will or may wish to do the following:

1. Seek medical care and ongoing evaluation
2. Take reasonable steps to avoid potential and identifiable risks to his or her own health and the health of his or her patients
3. Inform, as or when appropriate, relevant patients, administrators, or medical personnel

HIV AND HBV TESTING

Athletic trainers should follow federal, state, local, and institutional laws, regulations, and guidelines regarding HIV and HBV testing. Athletic trainers should, in appropriate practice settings and situations, find it advisable to educate or assist athletes with respect to the availability of testing.

HBV VACCINATIONS

Consistent with professional requirements and restrictions, athletic trainers should encourage HBV vaccinations for all employees at risk, in accordance with OSHA guidelines.

WITHHOLDING OF CARE AND DISCRIMINATION

NATA's policies and its Code of Ethics make it unethical to discriminate illegally on the basis of medical conditions.

Approved by the NATA Board of Directors
May 11, 1995

Bibliography

American Academy of Pediatrics. Human immunodeficiency virus (acquired immunodeficiency syndrome (AIDS) virus) in the athletic setting. *Pediatrics.* 1991;88:640-641.

American Medical Association, Department of HIV, Division of Health Science. *Digest of HIV/AIDS Policy.* Chicago, Ill: American Medical Association, Department of HIV; 1993:1-15.

American Medical Society of Sports Medicine and American Academy of Sports Medicine. Human immunodeficiency virus (HIV) and other blood-borne pathogens in sports. *American Journal of Sports Medicine.* In press.

Benson MT, ed. *NCAA Sports Medicine Handbook*; 1993:24-28.

Michigan Department of Public Health. Michigan recommendations on HBV-and/or HIV-infected health care workers. *Triad.* 1992;4:32-34.

Reprinted with permission from the NATA.

Medical Imaging and Special Diagnostic Procedures

Arthrography: A procedure involving the injection of a radiopaque medium into a joint. The joint is then passively moved through a range of motion while radiographs are taken. The image produced outlines the pathological status of soft tissue structures not seen on plain radiographs (e.g., meniscal tears, ligament tears).

Bone Scan: This procedure involves the injection of radioactive isotopes intravenously. A scan of the bone is then taken approximately 3 hours later. The bone scan displays increased uptakes of the isotopes at the site of injury or disease. Common pathologies seen may include fractures, tumors, abnormal growths, or infection.

Computed Tomography (CT scan): A process by which x-ray beams are projected through the patient and measured by a detector as they emerge. The CT scan moves across the body taking numerous measurements and provides for cross-sectional views in sagittal and coronal planes. These measurements are stored in a computer and reconstructed to produce a series of images. CT scans aid to reveal the extent of injuries to bone and soft tissue.

Diagnostic Arthroscopy: An invasive technique used to visually observe a joint and its structural components. Small incisions, called portals, are created to insert equipment such as cameras, lights, and various surgical tools. A saline solution is used to flush and distend the joint so as to provide for better visualization. The structures identified by the camera are able to be viewed via a television monitor. This allows for not only a diagnosis but also for any treatment that needs to be performed while the surgeon has access to the involved joint. Arthroscopic procedures are performed on a regular basis to joints such as the shoulder, elbow, wrist, hip, knee, and ankle.

Electromyography (EMG): The recognition and amplification of electrical signals that are produced by a voluntary muscle contraction. This technique utilizes needle-type electrodes that are anatomically placed over individual muscles. The electrical activity is then recorded graphically and displayed on an oscilloscope. EMG can be helpful in detecting peripheral nerve injuries or muscle denervation.

Fluoroscopy: Radiographic views are projected onto a fluorescent screen for immediate observation, thus providing a "live-action" view of the interior of the body. The advantage to this technique is that a clinician can examine a body part rather quickly as opposed to waiting for the development of film. In addition, a special piece of equipment referred to as a "spot-film device" can be used if a permanent record of the image is desired.

Magnetic Resonance Imaging (MRI): A noninvasive procedure utilized to assist with diagnosis of neurological or musculoskeletal injuries. A patient is placed in a magnetic field that allows for the body to emit electromagnetic waves. These waves are detected and transferred to a computer, all without the use of ionizing radiation. The computer constructs and provides images in sagittal, coronal, and oblique planes that clearly depict the anatomy and physiology of the body part being examined.

Myelography: A procedure in which a radiopaque contrast medium is injected into the intrathecal space via a lumbar puncture. Following the injection, the person undergoing this procedure is tilted on a tilt table until the medium flows to the desired area. Radiographs are then taken to identify the pattern outlined by the contrast medium and flow. The procedure may take 6–8 hours and the patient is instructed to lie flat for 24 hours following the procedure because symptoms of nausea have been found to be associated with this procedure as a result of fluid changes. The results of this test may reveal any distortion of the spinal cord or spinal dural sac that may be caused by herniated discs, cysts, or tumors.

Nerve Conduction Velocity Study: This type of test is used to assess the conduction velocity of either a motor or sensory nerve. Motor nerve conduction velocity studies involve the recording of a motor response from a superficially located skeletal muscle innervated by the peripheral nerve that is being studied. An oscilloscope is used to record the evoked action potentials of the muscle, which is figured into an equation to determine velocity. Assessment of a sensory nerve is similar to that of the motor nerve with the simple exception being that the skin is established as the site of stimulation as opposed to the muscle.

Surface electrodes are used to pick up signals of impulses. These tests are most often used to assess the integrity of peripheral nerves following an injury.

Plain Film Radiography: A technique commonly used to identify bone or joint disorders. Plain film radiography is also known as an "x ray," which is an abbreviation for x-radiation. The process itself involves an x-ray beam that is absorbed by various tissues in assorted degrees that eventually create a shadow on unexposed film. Tissue with a greater density such as bone has a greater absorption and creates a white image. The lesser the density of the tissue, the lesser the absorption, thus the darker the image on the film. Radiographs detect fractures, changes in bone density, bone irregularity, and changes in joint structure. Plain film radiography is one-dimensional.

Documentation Abbreviations

General Terms

$\bar{a}$	before, prior to
ad lib	as desired
AMA	against medical advice
A or ant	anterior
AP	anterior/posterior
BID	twice daily
bilat	bilateral
BP	blood pressure
bpm	beats per minute
$\bar{c}$	with
c/c	chief complaint
c/o	complaints of
D/C or DC	discharge/discontinue
DTR	deep tendon relex
Dx	diagnosis
F/♀	female

FH	family history
Fx	fracture
H&P	history and physical
HEP	home exercise program
Htn	hypertension
Hx	history
Ⓛ	left
LE	lower extremity
LOC	loss of consciousness
M/♂	male
max	maximum
min	minimum/minute
mod	moderate
NPO	nothing by mouth
p̄	after
per	by
PMH	part medical history
PO	by mouth
post	after/posterior
PRE	progressive resistive exercise
PRN	as needed
pt	patient
PTA	prior to admission
q	every
qd	every day
QID	four times a day
qod	every other day
q2h	every 2 hours
Ⓡ	right
R/O	rule out
RTC	return to clinic
Rx	treatment
s̄	without
sob	shortness of breath
s/p	status post
stat	immediately
Sx	symptoms
TID	three times a day
UE	upper extremity
UTI	urinary tract infection
VO/vo	verbal order
VS	vital signs
w/c	wheelchair

WFC	within functional limits
WNL	within normal limits
y/o	year old

Symbols

>	greater than
<	less than
↑	increase
↓	decrease
®	to follow
1°	primary/first degree
2°	secondary/due to/second degree
3°	tertiary/third degree
@	at
Δ	change
~	approximately
♀	female
♂	male

Rehabilitation Abbreviations

ADL	activities of daily living
AFO	ankle foot orthosis
amb	ambulation
HVPGS	hi-volt pulsed galvanic stimulation
EMS	electrical muscle stimulation
Ex	exercise
Ind	independent
x	times
ms	muscle
hemi	hemiplegia
PNF	proprioceptive neuromuscular facilitation
FEMS	functional electrical muscle stimulation
TENS	transcutaneous electrical nerve stimulation
NDT	neuro developmental training
HP	hot pack
US	ultrasound
M/mas	massage
MMT	manual muscle test
HUM	hot pack, ultrasound, massage
ROM	range of motion

Dep   dependent
WC   wheelchair

Abbreviations that are Best Written Out When Documentation Is to be Provided to Outside Payers

AROM   active range of motion
AAROM   active assistive range of motion
ASROM   assistive range of motion
PROM   passive range of motion
AE   above elbow
AK   above knee
BE   below elbow
BK   below knee
NWB   non-weight bearing
PWB   partial weight bearing
TDWB   touch down weight bearing
WB   weight bearing

Muscle Test Grading

Grade	Value	Movement
5	Normal	Complete ROM against gravity with maximal resistance
4	Good	Complete ROM against gravity with moderate resistance
3+	Fair+	Complete ROM against gravity with minimal resistance
3	Fair	Complete ROM against gravity
3-	Fair-	Incomplete ROM against gravity
2+	Poor+	Initiates motion against gravity
2	Poor	Complete ROM, gravity reduced
2-	Poor-	Initiates ROM, gravity reduced
1	Trace	Evidence of slight contraction, no joint movement
0	Zero	No contraction seen or palpated

Glossary of Terms

Accreditation: The process of recognizing standards that are met and maintained within an institution that would enable a person to receive a certificate or registration in a certain domain.

Acquired Immune Deficiency Syndrome (AIDS): A terminal virus that leads to a destruction of the immune system.

Administrative policies: Policies set forth for those working in the same facility or who are employed under the same management.

Advertising: Paid, nonpersonal communications by business firms, nonprofit organizations, and individuals who are identified in their advertising message and who hope to inform or persuade members of particular audiences.

American Physical Therapy Association (APTA): The national membership group for physical therapists and physical therapist assistants.

Asthma: Bronchospasms as a result of hypersensitivity to the trachea and/or bronchi.

Business plan: A plan that explains the business' future revenue and expense predictions, including overall operations, profits, and losses.

C Corporation: A form of a corporation in which the company pays taxes at a corporate rate.

Capitation: A fixed, per capita method of payment to a provider for health services over a specific period of time for each person served, regardless of the amount of service rendered.

Certification: A form of regulation restricting performance functions to specific individuals or professions.

Chronic bronchitis: Inflammation of the bronchi resulting in an irritable and productive cough.

Chronic Obstructive Pulmonary Disease (COPD): A condition whereby exchange of gases in the respiratory system is ineffective.

Clinical/Industrial/Corporate Athletic Trainers' Committee (C/I/C Committee): A subsection of the NATA.

Continuing Education Unit (CEU): Learning opportunities made available that may lead to professional growth.

Corporation: A business organization in which ownership is divided into shares of stock. Corporations have perpetual life and the principal stock owners of the corporation face only a limited liability.

Co-payment: A cost sharing whereby the insured member pays a specific flat fee per unit of service at the time selected services are rendered.

Departmental policies: Policies designed to affect a specific group of people performing different tasks than other groups within the same organization.

Diabetes mellitus: A condition resulting from inability to produce or distribute insulin.

Effectiveness: The extent to which benefits achievable under optimal conditions of care are actually achieved in clinical practice.

Efficacy: The probability of benefit to individuals in a defined population from a medical technology applied for a given medical problem under ideal conditions of use.

Emphysema: A destruction of bronchioles and alveoli via a weakening or rupturing resulting in an inflation of the lungs.

Epilepsy: A temporary disturbance of electrical impulses of the brain.

Evaluation: The process of comparing objectives, strategies, and goals with actual results. This information should have both qualitative and quantitative data.

Exclusive Provider Organization (EPO): A more rigid type of health plan that requires the insured to use only designated providers or forfeit reimbursement altogether.

Exemption: A political process through which a state legislature recognizes that functions of an identified, though unregulated, profession duplicate those of a licensed profession.

External environment assessment: Provides a picture of the external opportunities, threats, and constraints that may have an impact on the intended program and/or services.

Fee-for-service: Traditional method of paying for medical services whereby a health care provider bills for each encounter or service rendered.

Franchise tax: A type of tax in which cost is based upon a company's authorized capital stock.

Gatekeeper: A primary care physician who provides the initial evaluation and makes appropriate referrals when necessary.

Grand mal seizure: A type of seizure involving violent, shaking convulsions, and a loss of consciousness.

Health Maintenance Organization (HMO): An organization that provides a wide range of comprehensive health care services for a specified member group, at a fixed rate.

Hodgkin's disease: A virus producing impaired lymphocyte characterized by exacerbations and remissions.

Human Immunodeficiency Virus (HIV): A virus recognized as the causative agent for AIDS, which leads to a deteriorating immune system and promotes increased susceptibility to infection and illness.

Hypertension: Blood pressure above normal limits.

Indemnity health plans: Plans that offer selected coverages within a set framework of fee schedules, limitations, and exclusions. Reimbursement is made after carriers review claims.

Industrial setting: Nontraditional location typically consisting of corporations, companies, or employees whose main work-related task is not of the athletic or sporting nature.

Infectious mononucleosis: A self-limiting lymphoproliferative disease caused by the Epstein-Barr Virus.

Interdepartmental policies: Policies designed to organize the actions of different disciplines that may be working to achieve the same common goal.

Internal environment assessment: The analyzing and defining of the factors within the organization that may help or hinder development and growth of a program or service.

Licensure: Strongest form of regulation for a profession via the establishment of standards of practice.

Macro-marketing: A social process that directs an economy's flow of goods and services from producer to consumer in a way that effectively matches supply and demand and accomplishes the objectives of society.

Macro objectives: Planning process to establish broad, overall objectives to set performance targets and measure progress.

Managed care: Health care systems that integrate the financing and delivery of appropriate health care services to covered individuals by arrangements with selected providers to furnish a comprehensive set of health care services.

Market segment: A relatively homogeneous group of customers who will respond to a marketing mix in a similar way.

Marketing: Process of planning and executing the conception, pricing, promotion, and distribution of ideas, goods, services, organizations, and events to create exchanges that satisfy individual and organizational objectives.

Marketing mix: The controllable variable that the company puts together to satisfy a target group. The four plus two "Ps" product, price, place, promotion, patient relations, and pride.

Mission: General statement of organizational purposes.

Mission statement: A statement or number of statements that define the goals and philosophies of an organization or department.

National Athletic Trainers' Association (NATA): The national membership group of the athletic trainers.

Nontraditional setting: A physical therapy clinic, hospital-based clinic, industrial setting, or personal fitness training.

Occupational burnout: A syndrome of physical and emotional exhaustion involving the development of both a negative self-concept and a poor or negative attitude toward an individual's job.

Outcomes assessment: A systematic method used for measuring the effects of an intervention.

Outcomes measurements: Observation of an individual's course of medical treatment within a specific time period. Outcomes typically link patient's satisfaction and health status with clinical measurements and associated cost factors.

Partnership: A business organization in which two or more people under a contractual agreement are co-owners of the company.

Petit mal seizure: A type of seizure consisting of short duration, low level twitches that rarely involve a loss of consciousness.

Point of Service (POS): A managed care plan that encourages the use of network providers, but permits insured individuals to choose providers outside the plan.

Policy: A definite course or method of action selected from alternatives and in light of given conditions to guide and determine present and future decisions.

Preferred Provider Organization (PPO): An organization whereby a third party payer contracts with a group of preferred providers who furnish services at lower than customary fees.

Primary care provider: An individual who provides the initial care to a person seeking medical attention.

Procedure: The act or series of steps that are used to carry out a policy.

Promotion: Function of informing, persuading, and influencing the buyer's purchase decision.

Psoriasis: A chronic, hortatory skin disorder that presents with red, scaly patches.

Raynaud's disease: An arterial disorder decreasing blood flow to the fingers and toes as a result of a vasospasm brought upon by exposure to cold environments or stressful circumstances.

Quality assessment: The measurement of the technical and interpersonal aspects of medical care.

Quality of care: That component of the difference between efficacy and effectiveness that can be attributed to care providers, taking account of the environment in which they work.

Registration: Least restrictive form of regulation of a profession as it merely serves to list or identify practitioners of a single type.

Regulation: The process of enacting a rule or law in an attempt to bring order, method, or uniformity to an issue.

Reserved name: By reserving or registering a facility's name protects the name (or every similar name) from being used by other parties.

Risk management: A plan that the clinical owner makes in order to minimize potential loss.

Scope of practice: A set of parameters that when combined together define the legal capabilities of a profession or professional.

Secondary care provider: An individual who renders services, equipment, or testing procedures that are not readily available at the primary care level.

Segmenting: An aggregating process that clusters people with similar needs into a market segment (athletic people).

Sickle cell disease: A hemolytic hereditary disorder associated with structural defect of the oxygen carrying hemoglobin of the red blood cells.

Sole proprietorship: The simplest form of a business organization in which the entire business is owned by one individual.

Strategic planning process: A method in which a project can be organized and evaluated by pulling together staff and others in the area with similar interests in the project.

Strategic planing team: A team that can be made up of anyone you deemed necessary to make this plan pull together and come into fruition. People in the area who may be interested in the outcome, if in some way that will also benefit them (win/win), can be evaluated.

Sub-S Corporation: A form of a corporation in which personal profits or losses of the corporation are reflected on the individual stockholders personal income tax, thereby taxed at their personal income tax rate.

Target market: A fairly similar group of customers to whom a company wishes to appeal. This might be the more athletic health consumer.

Tertiary care provider: The incorporation of a facility that has the capability to provide both primary and secondary levels of care in order to service a community.

Traditional setting: Athletic training room or department.

Traumatogens: A source of biomechanical stress stemming from job-related demands that exceed an individual's capabilities.

Utilization review: A process designed to evaluate health care on the basis of appropriateness, necessity, and quality.

INDEX